Skin Cleanse

THE SIMPLE, ALL-NATURAL PROGRAM
FOR CLEAR, CALM, HAPPY SKIN

Adina Grigore

HARPER WAVE

An Imprint of HarperCollins*Publishers*

HarperCollins books may be purchased for educational, business, or sales promotional use. For information, please e-mail the Special Markets Department at SPsales@harpercollins.com.

FIRST EDITION

Designed by Renato Stanisic
Illustrations by Libby VanderPloeg

Library of Congress Cataloging-in-Publication Data

Grigore, Adina.
Skin cleanse ˙: the simple, all-natural program for clear, calm, happy skin / Adina Grigore. — First edition.
pages cm
ISBN 978-0-06-233255-4 (hardback)
1. Skin—Care and hygiene. 2. Nutrition. 3. Detoxification (Health) 4. Self-care, Health. I. Title.
RL87.G73 2015
613'.488—dc23

2014044382

15 16 17 18 19   OV/RRD   10 9 8 7 6 5 4 3 2 1

DEDICATED TO YOU, BECAUSE YOU'RE AWESOME.

CONTENTS

INTRODUCTION

've been sensitive my whole life. I have a sensitive belly and sensitive skin and I cry at sad commercials. When I was little, I was plagued by mysterious stomachaches after every meal and headaches that had no apparent cause. By the time I was thirteen, my parents rotated picking me up from school and taking me to different doctors to try to figure out what was wrong. No one ever could, and my symptoms kept getting worse. I moved to New York City for college and by that time I was scared of every food; I was getting migraines every week; and I was covered in itchy, rashy skin. As you can imagine, it was pretty awesome.

After I graduated, I went back to school to study holistic health and nutrition. I also became interested in fitness and exercise science and got a job as a personal trainer at a local gym. By that point, I had learned enough about different nutritional theories that I was able to calm my stomachaches and migraines by making small tweaks to my diet. It felt really empowering to be able to fix myself when doctors had only been scratching their heads and prescribing me pills. Helping people take better care of themselves and teaching them how to be healthy all on their own—without having to pay expensive "experts"—became a passion of mine.

As for my skin? Nothing had changed.

I was in my early twenties, and I was dealing with a horrific trifecta: constant breakouts; itchy, dry scalp; and an undiagnosable body rash that wouldn't go away. I was already using two different heavy-duty medicated treatments for my breakouts and rash, and my dermatologist had just given me a new shampoo for my scalp. But when I started to use it, I quickly and painfully realized that my new shampoo made my leg rash freak out.

So I did what any person driven completely insane would do: I started showering upside down. Normal, right? I'm not kidding. I would flip my head over to wash my hair and rinse really well, to make sure that the suds from the shampoo wouldn't drip onto my itchy legs.

Luckily, it didn't take too many showers for me to realize how completely ridiculous my skin-care routine had become. I had studied holistic health and nutrition for years and had learned so much about my internal health, but I had somehow managed to ignore my skin completely. I was treating it as if it wasn't a part of my well-being at all. I had finally gotten healthy enough to need a doctor only rarely, but I was addicted to dermatologists. As I said before, I was on actual prescription medications for my skin problems. I was like an addict, but instead of being hooked on pills, I was hooked on creams, baby.

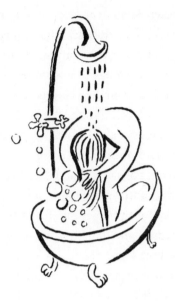

Those miserable, painful, upside-down showers were my rock bottom. I just felt so ugly and itchy and frustrated, and I couldn't do it anymore. I couldn't keep using these products that were meant to help but were turning my life into a nightmare. So I quit. I stopped using every single skin-care product and medication. Cold turkey. I thought to myself, *Maybe I'll be single forever and people will avoid standing next to me, but at least I won't be itchy anymore.* It was my last, desperate attempt at finding some relief.

And, shockingly, relief did come. It was pretty much instantaneous. That whole first day of using no products whatsoever, all of my symptoms improved. And the next day, I felt even better. Every day, I waited for proof that this was too good to be true. How was it possible no one had told me to try this miraculous cure?

Then came the research. Reluctantly, the first place I went to was my kitchen cabinet. I knew all about holistic health and nutrition and the amazing things that eating good food could do for my body, and I wondered if it was possible to use on my skin the same ingredients I was eating. But if it was soooo great, why wasn't everyone doing it? I tested my theory anyway, and watched as my rash improved after using olive oil—straight up extra-virgin olive oil, the same kind you use as salad dressing. I tried shaving my legs with coconut oil (after even going so far as to peel the moisture strips off my razors because they were making my rash worse) and didn't get razor burn for maybe the first time in my whole life. I rinsed my scalp with apple cider vinegar and noticed that not only was my scalp not itchy the next day, but my cheeks were rosy and clearer, too. So then I put it straight on my face, and voilà! Breakouts gone.

If this sounds completely insane to you, you are not alone. But think about it: we've been spending *years* and *years* shifting our conversation about food. I work with clients to teach them how to eat healthy and work out to feel better. They already know to think of good food and fitness as medicine. Yet somehow this idea still has not crossed over into our conversations about skin care. Ingredients like preservatives and artificial chemicals that have become hugely infamous in food do not have the same reputations when they are in our face washes. And most simply and most importantly, no one really talks about how the olive oil that lowers our cholesterol and provides our bodies with healthy fat is the same exact olive oil that can cure psoriasis and fight stretch marks.

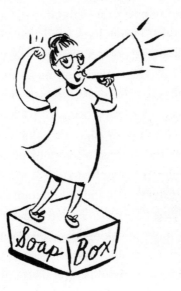

So, awkwardly, painfully, and sometimes upside down, I found my mission: to tell you and every human on the planet that healthy skin must be nourished in the exact same way as a healthy body—and with the exact same ingredients.

I launched an organization called Sprout Wellness dedicated to this idea and taught workshops about what I had learned. I developed DIY skin-care recipes and gave long speeches about the magical, skin-calming powers hidden in your kitchen cabinet. I eventually turned those recipes into a full line of products called S.W. Basics ("S.W." stands for "Sprout Wellness," so that our company never forgets its roots in education and wellness). I still can't get over the fact that S.W. Basics products—which are still made using my original DIY recipes—are now sold in boutiques and retail chains all over the world.

To this day, my favorite thing to do is work one-on-one with clients and talk to people about the changes I made that gave me clear skin. Through my work and the work we do at S.W. Basics, thousands of people have started ditching their junky skin-care products and cleaning up their routines.

My ultimate goal is to get everyone to think of mainstream skin-care products like they think of packaged food: full of preservatives, unnecessary ingredients, and nasty chemicals. I want to lower the average number of products you use on your skin each day from twelve to one or two. To vastly reduce the even scarier number of individual ingredients the average woman is applying to her skin each day from hundreds to just a handful. To push the skin-care industry to get rid of the chemicals in their products that have been linked to cancer, reproductive disorders, asthma, and severe allergies. To make you understand that most of what you have been told and sold is not true, and the ability to have healthy, happy skin is totally and completely in your hands.

In baby steps, though. I don't want you to feel as if you *have* to stop doing anything you like, but I want to help you not *need* any of it. I want you to feel like an expert by the end of this book. An expert on *you*, *your* body, and *your* skin. To feel like you're the boss and in control and, best of all, like you can stop stressing over how to have good skin once and for all. How nice would that be? The best part is that it's not even going to be that hard. This entire book is about things that you intuitively know. You're going to read through everything and think, *Ohhhhh, duh.* I'm a testament to the fact that you can find out what's best for you with a little bit of guidance, and so are all of the people I've worked with, and all of the people I've never met who have figured out that going back to the basics is the best thing you can do for yourself.

So, here's how it's gonna go. We're going to discuss why your skin is already amazing all on its own, before you ever put any products on it. I mean, no one else is saying that, definitely not the antiaging-serum and zit-cream commercials. But it's about time they did. Your skin is a truly incredible and efficient organ, and we're going to show it the respect and care it deserves. Next, I'm going to teach you how to put your skin's health and overall well-being into context so you can get a big-picture view of the many factors that affect it. The tiny little "skin type" boxes that we assign ourselves to don't really help us achieve healthy skin—they're just helping us buy more products. So I'm going to show you how much more complex you are than marketers would have you believe. Then, we're going to talk a *lot* about food, because a clean diet is the number one way to have a lifetime of great skin. We're also going to talk about your products and unveil the dirty underworld of the cosmetic-industrial complex. After that, I'm going to offer you a little challenge to get you back on track, and finally, we're going to make some beautiful DIY products together.

Sound good? Great! This book is the program that I offer to people who work with me because they're frustrated and fed up and want answers. I hope you find all of your answers in here, too!

Skin Cleanse

CHAPTER 1

YOUR AMAZING SKIN

Here's what you've probably learned about your skin from a lifetime of reading lady magazines and watching television:

Zits are the worst thing your skin can do to you, and if you get them, people will no longer talk to you, they'll only talk to your zits—and they'll be horrified. To get rid of zits, you have to *stop them before they start*™. Once you've taken care of the zits, you have to start worrying about your collagen production and your skin's elasticity. If you don't, you will get wrinkles and signs of aging way before you should, which is basically anytime ever, even if you're 150 years old. If that's not enough, you also have these huge ugly things called pores, and you should do your absolute best to shrink and hide them. You need to keep out of the sun at all costs, wear multiple layers of sunscreen at all times, and wear long sleeves and a hat, even in the summer. Above all, your skin is helpless without you. The only way you can stop the zits, stop the aging, up the collagen and elasticity, prevent sun damage, and minimize those ugly pores is to use products. Lots and lots of them.

Think about it. Of all the information you have about your skin, how much of it came from someone trying to sell you something? In what other context have you ever heard the words *collagen* or *pigmentation* or *rejuvenation*? When you close your eyes and imagine the layers that make up your skin, do you see a bright, cartoonish illustration with some squiggly lines and polka dots differentiating the layers? Can you hear a voiceover describing some face wash that is going to "penetrate" your pores to give you a "deep clean"? Gross.

And you probably don't even know what a lot of those words really mean. What, exactly, is a pore? What's the difference between your dermis and your epidermis? What is collagen, and why is losing it so terrifying? Most of us, even if we're experts in skin-care products, know very little about our actual skin. Why? Because we haven't been properly educated. We've been sold a bunch of catchy slogans and advertising graphics.

THE BASICS

So, let's take a look at the facts.

Your skin is your largest organ. Wait, wait, let me back up. Your skin is an *organ*. Like your heart, or your liver. Meaning, it is a specialized set of tissues that works together to perform necessary biological functions. Your skin keeps water inside your body, regulates your temperature, protects your internal organs from the outside world, turns sunlight into vitamin D (a nutrient you need to stay alive), and flushes toxins out of your body. You are made up of almost ten pounds, or twenty square feet, of skin.

Your skin is part of a group of organs known as the integumentary system, which also includes your hair, nails, and sweat glands. Most of us think that our skin operates completely independently from other systems in the body, such as the digestive system, endocrine system, nervous system, and so on. We treat the skin as if it's just a shield protecting our insides from the outside world—a shield we want to keep looking beautiful, glowing, and smooth, but a shield all the same. The truth is, your skin belongs to the incredible, interconnected whole that is your body. Its health is as much a part of your general well-being as the health of your brain, your liver, or your heart.

· · · ·

So let's take a moment to understand and appreciate this outer covering of yours!

Your **epidermis** is the top layer of your skin, and it contains four types of skin cells. Keratinocytes produce keratin, a fibrous protein that guards your body against heat, bacteria, and chemicals. Melanocytes produce melanin, which is responsible for the color of your skin and protects you from the sun by absorbing UV light. Langerhans cells function like the immune system of your skin by helping produce antibodies that fight infection. And then there are Merkel cells, which connect to your nerve cells and allow you to experience the sensation of touch. Your epidermis is about a tenth of a millimeter thick, except on your palms and feet, which are layered with an extra two millimeters of cushioning. Because, you know, they work pretty hard.

The **dermis** is right underneath your epidermis, and it is made up of proteins you've heard of many times: elastin and collagen. They make your skin strong, stretchy, and, as you may have guessed, elastic. When you cut your skin, your dermis produces extra collagen to fill and heal the wound. Your dermis also produces hyaluronic acid, a chemical that helps hold hydration in the skin, making you look youthful. The constant activity in your dermis is what we correlate with "healthy" skin: it's doing all of the behind-the-scenes work to make your skin look soft and vibrant.

Beneath those two layers is your **subcutaneous fat**, which, as its name suggests, is a layer of fat that connects the nerves from your dermis and epidermis to the rest of your body, while also protecting your insides with a really sexy cushion.

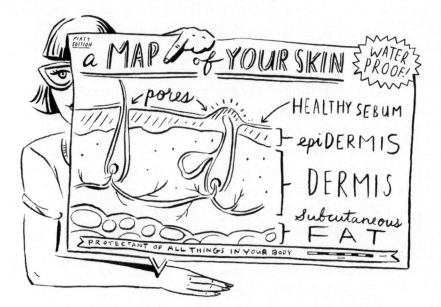

Skin-care commercials probably don't want you to know this, but your epidermis, dermis, and subcutaneous fat actually work together to give your skin a set of natural superpowers.

Skin is capable of regenerating itself. You are constantly shedding dead skin cells (no big deal, just 30,000 to 40,000 every minute) so that healthy, fresh ones produced by the epidermis can replace them. This is happening regardless of what you apply topically. And as you get older, this regenerative process slows down, no matter how great your plastic surgeon is. With age, your body not only produces less of these proteins, but their quality also diminishes. This is why your skin changes. Age spots happen (so does gray hair) because your melanin weakens over time. Wrinkles and sagging skin are the result of your collagen and elastin becoming stiffer and more brittle, making your skin crease (or wrinkle) and become less plump (sag). These are just normal results of aging. But here's the secret: the healthier you are internally, the longer you can produce youthful skin cells.

Your skin is also a powerful barrier. Thanks to a sealant created by keratinocytes, our skin is nearly waterproof. When you hold water in your hand, it doesn't soak in. (The only part of your body that isn't waterproof is the inside of your mouth.) But this barrier is not impenetrable, which is why your fingers get pruney after being in the pool too long. The same is true for other chemicals you put on your skin. Absorption does occur, and most of what soaks in will make it to your bloodstream and circulatory system, sometimes within seconds. The amount of any substance you absorb depends on the level of your exposure: how much, for how long, and how often.

Another amazing property of skin is that it is naturally self-protecting. The oil that your skin produces is a good thing. It's called sebum. It keeps your hair from drying out, it stops too much water from evaporating off your skin, it keeps your skin soft, and, perhaps most importantly, it kills bacteria. In other words, it is not an evil substance that only makes you break out. Sebum also creates what is called an acid mantle, which neutralizes the effects of chemicals and environmental toxins by keeping your skin slightly acidic. This is crucial because the pH of your skin has a lot to do with its health. Skin that is too alkaline will become dry and itchy, while too much acidity will make you prone to inflammation and breakouts. Most outside contaminants make us more alkaline, so your acid mantle keeps them from throwing you out of balance. You've been taught to think of "oily skin" as the worst thing in the world, but that's confusing the issue. Your skin's oil is important, and you shouldn't think of it as an enemy.

Get ready for another shocking idea those skin-care commercials would never tell you: your skin cleans itself . . . whether or not you use a fancy exfoliant. One of the ways the integumentary system works with the body's other organs is that waste toxins are expelled through sweat, and your skin contains a whole ecosystem of healthy bacteria that are responsible for eliminating them. This ecosystem is called your **skin flora**, and not only does it get rid of the bad stuff in your sweat, it's constantly fighting outside organisms to keep them from entering your body. The reason you stink when you sweat is because the bacteria on your skin is eating the toxins in your sweat. It may sound super-gross, but it's actually kind of incredible when you think about it. In addition to the barrier your skin already creates against invaders, this army of bacteria provides a second defense system.

None of these natural superpowers require you to use skin-care products. When you stay out of your skin's way by maintaining a good diet and a healthy lifestyle, it has the ability to function as its own mini–immune system, fighting invaders like dirt and bacteria. It can protect itself in the face of the elements, and it has the power to keep itself in check. The only time it stops working efficiently is when its natural balance gets disrupted: hormone changes can cause an overproduction of sebum, toxins cause an overproduction of skin flora, and so on.

So, don't you think your skin deserves some love? We spend a lot of time resenting how much attention we have to pay to our skin, and how much time and money it can take. But think about how important it is to your body and how many different functions it serves. On top of that, it's exposed to all of the horrors of the world: sunburns, ski slopes, hot tubs, hot tubs on ski slopes, a sharp blade that removes your hair over and over, face paint you put on every single day, and chemical products that are the technological equivalent of your car's gasoline.

It's a wonder our skin even puts up with us.

Skin is also a window to what's happening inside your body. Just because you topically soothe its symptoms does not mean you've corrected the issues causing them in the first place. Think about it this way: we know that eating oatmeal helps to lower cholesterol naturally and, therefore, may help to prevent heart disease. But smearing oatmeal on the outside of your heart wouldn't exactly have the same effect, right? In other words, it is not the $300 serum that "anti-ages" you, it's how you treat the inside of your body that ages or anti-ages your skin.

But unlike your other organs, your skin is totally exposed! It's not neatly tucked inside your body and protected. In fact, it is *the* protector. It is taking all of the hits so that the rest of your organs don't have to. This makes the way you treat it massively important. Your skin is getting nourished or harmed from the inside, *and* nourished or harmed from the outside! So if you expose your skin to poison ivy, you will hurt it. And if you eat a food you are allergic to, you might break out in a rash that looks and feels something like a poison ivy reaction.

SKIN TROUBLES

How often do you visit your dermatologist? In my experience, most people don't go nearly enough, if at all. You get regular physicals for your insides, so why not for your outsides? First of all, skin cancer is incredibly curable if it is caught early, so that should be reason enough to have an annual appointment. But a visit to the dermatologist is also a way to check in on the health of your skin and, therefore, the health of your insides, with a *professional*. (Meaning, not your eyebrow threader or bikini waxer.) At the very least, a dermatologist is going to remind you that you're not taking care of your skin and that you'd better start, fast. I'm all for that.

That said, I get frustrated when clients tell me they leave their dermatologists with a new prescription every time they visit. Prescriptions aren't the answer, or, at least, the only answer, for the vast majority of people who are dealing with skin issues. I've seen people experience the same symptoms over and over again and not be able to get answers from anywhere, including their dermatologists' prescription pads. At my nutrition school, skin ailments weren't on the syllabus at all, and it was only after dealing with my own chronic skin problems that I made the connection between my overall health and my incurable rashes. In my experience of talking to frustrated people who say exactly the same things time and again, medications have never been able to solve all of their ailments, and, in some cases, they've spawned new ones. Sadly, that's partly because the science of skin care isn't quite as advanced as we want it to be, or assume it is.

Don't believe me? Well, even dermatology isn't able to offer concrete causes of—and solutions for—many skin conditions. Here are a few examples:

Acne results from your pores getting clogged by dead skin cells and too much sebum, and then aggravated by bacteria. The reason you get acne as a teenager is because your oil glands are growing in size and producing more oil than your skin actually needs. This also happens when you're pregnant. According to the science, acne *may* also be related to hormones, or to skin flora, or even to inflammation in the body. The treatments recommended for acne by the American Academy of Dermatology (AAD) include antibiotics, birth control, lasers, and chemical peels.[1]

Psoriasis is what we call it when your epidermis produces too many cells, which leads to a condition that feels scaly but is really like having too much skin. Psoriasis is a result of a struggling immune system—possibly you had a virus in your past and your system has not completely recovered . . . or possibly not. According to the AAD, "Scientists are still trying to learn everything that happens inside the body to cause psoriasis."[2]

Dermatitis is itchy, red skin that can either be caused by something internal (atopic dermatitis, or eczema) or from something that touches your skin and aggravates it (contact dermatitis). The reaction following exposure to poison ivy is contact dermatitis. Lots of different things can cause contact dermatitis, including soap. And water. Incidents of both types of dermatitis are on the rise, and no scientific cause has been found.

Eczema, or atopic dermatitis, doesn't really mean anything. It's a catch-all term that means, very simply, skin ailment. A million unexplained symptoms have been grouped under eczema. You should think of it more as code for "Something weird is going on with your skin and we don't really know what it is." The AAD, again: "Doctors don't really know why some kids and adults get eczema, and others don't."[3]

Rosacea is bright-red flushing of the skin on your face. As you may have guessed, scientifically, no cause has been linked other than inflammation and possibly bad bacteria in the gut. (Amen to that discovery, at least!) Rosacea can make your skin bumpy and swollen, and it makes you extremely sensitive to many topical ingredients.

Hyperpigmentation is when your skin has a darker pigment, or color, because you are producing too much melanin. Hyperpigmentation has been linked to hormones, viruses, too much sun exposure, and (here it is again) inflammation.

Sunburn. Okay so maybe we know what causes this one. But the interesting thing about all the hate we have for the sun is that a *mild* amount of sun to completely bare skin is not only significantly better for synthesizing vitamin D, it also forces your skin cells to produce more melanin (that's why your skin gets darker), which actually ends up protecting you from the sun and from future sunburns. So overexposure is bad, but a little natural light on your skin is actually good for you. Also, this is, amazingly, the one area that science has found a solid correlation with diet: the better you eat, the less likely you are to get burned.[4]

So while your dermatologist is definitely your friend and ally when it comes to calming the symptoms of chronic, sometimes miserable skin conditions, I believe it's a mistake to rely too much on a symptom-soothing approach. Hopefully, you noticed some of the common denominators in all of those vague definitions of various ailments: things like hormone imbalance, inflammation, and a struggling immune system.

When you think in those terms, it's easy to feel as if the health of your skin is out of your control, and only a cream or spot treatment can help. But hormones can be more or less balanced, inflammation can be made better or worse, and an immune system can be improved or weakened based on what you eat and how you treat your body. The way to get healthy skin is to create a healthy body, and you get a healthy body by making smart food and lifestyle choices.

YOU JUST CAN'T THINK of your products and medications as the one and only way to take care of your skin. If you have a recurring skin problem, it is almost definitely the result of something going on internally. If you heal it topically, it will be a temporary solution, a bandage. Until you correct whatever is causing the flare-up internally, you are simply masking the symptom. In some ways, it's amazing that topical ingredients can help to heal an inside problem from the outside. It's so cool that a little aloe will relieve your itchy or burned skin, a dab of vinegar will even your skin tone, and a spot of baking soda will diminish a zit. But none of these will soothe your upset digestive system, your stressed-out nerves, or your depleted blood cells.

RETHINKING SKIN HEALTH

The fact that we pay attention to our skin only when it freaks out is a problem. Dermatologists, like other doctors, can help us one symptom at a time, which means that, to take *real* care of our skin, we have to take *real* care of our bodies generally.

And what do I mean by that? Let me introduce you to a concept I call your *ideal everyday health.*

Ideal everyday health is the best *you* you can be. It's not trying to look like Megan Fox or Channing Tatum. Instead, your ideal everyday health is completely unique to your background, your lifestyle, and your diet. If you're a sixty-year-old Korean woman who's been active her whole life, your ideal everyday health is going to be very different from that of a thirty-year-old Irish woman who hates exercise, or a sixteen-year-old black girl feeling the stress of teenagerhood. Each of us can be healthier or less healthy in our unique circumstances, and, honestly, it's not our doctor's job to ensure our ideal everyday health—it's *ours.*

Which brings me back to how all of those advertisers and articles have taught you to think about your skin. I call it *skin shame.* You are paranoid, obsessive, and ashamed of your skin every waking minute of every day, right? Who could blame you? And what's worse, hating yourself and being stressed just perpetuates the problems, causing you to pile on too many products full of chemicals. Women hate their skin even when it's perfect and glowing. I'll tell you a secret: none of my clients ever really have the skin they think they see in the mirror. But as far back as they can remember, they've been told they do. And you have, too. We all have. This book is about stopping skin shame.

Don't worry, you can keep going to the dermatologist, keep getting facials, keep using products, keep reading those lady magazines, keep living the life you want. But I want you to walk away from this book feeling calmer about your skin and more in control of it. I'm here to give you the skin-care lesson you should've gotten a long time ago. By nourishing your skin from the inside, with the kind of healthy, individualized diet I'm going to help you develop for yourself, and from the outside, with the easy, gentle DIY products I'll teach you how to make, you'll discover that you actually already have the amazing skin you've always wanted.

CHAPTER 2

YOU ARE WHAT YOUR GREAT-GRANDMOTHER ATE

Nine times out of ten, when new clients come to me looking for answers about their skin, they bring a self-diagnosis with them. Maybe they've convinced themselves they have a gluten intolerance, even though their doctor says they don't, or perhaps they're positive their hormones are out of whack or that everything wrong with them is a result of stress—but what can they possibly do about stress? And—ugh—don't even get them started on their oily T-zones . . . that's like a whole thing, too.

Here's the problem: people believe that everything they've ever heard or read about skin or diet applies to their individual bodies. When they hear that gluten is "bad" for them, they begin to see "gluten-intolerance" symptoms. When they hear that stress and hormones can negatively affect the skin, every pimple becomes a sign of being overstressed and hormonal. I appreciate people trying to educate themselves about their health, but this outlook gives people skin hypochondria. Every food and bodily process is suddenly viewed with suspicion, and they get a kind of throw-your-hands-in the-air resignation that good skin isn't even within their control.

Additionally, the easy, one-size-fits-all self-diagnosis isn't helpful because it doesn't actually help you get to the bottom of what is going on with your skin. Hormones act up, yes, but their effects can be made worse or better through lifestyle choices. Same with stress. It can be handled well or poorly. Gluten may not be your friend, but chances are, eating bread isn't the worst thing you are doing to your skin. Women with clear, healthy skin are not Paleo-eating stress-free robots who never get their periods. Skin is just like any other organ in the body; it is only as healthy as the rest of you.

THE WHOLE PICTURE

In order to really understand what's going on with your skin, you need to look at the whole picture of who you are. Your health is *your* health. Until you tune into you, into what makes your *particular* body your own, you cannot attribute one blanket cause to your symptoms. So get away from Google and WebMD. They are not your friends.

We're going to look at the three main factors that do affect your skin: background, lifestyle, and diet. These three elements are exactly what I mean when I say "the whole picture" of who you are. Where you came from, where your parents came from, where their parents came from—that's your background. Where you live now, what you do for a living, how you spend your free time, your fitness level, your habits, and the overall state of your health—that makes up your lifestyle today. How you eat now, how you ate five years ago, how you ate growing up—that's your diet. When you understand how these three areas relate to one another, you can have good skin almost all of the time. When you ignore or cause an imbalance in one of these areas, you will not. It's as simple as that. (But it's almost never just as simple as "I'm stressed" or "I'm hormonal," and, sorry, ladies, it's almost never "just gluten.")

Before we go any further, I want you to take five or ten minutes and answer a few questions. Write them down if you want, but it's not a pop quiz. I won't ask you to show your work. I just want you to have your individual background at the front of your mind before we drill down into more details.

1. Think about your genetic background. What is your ethnicity? Is it related to where you currently live? (For instance, if your family is Puerto Rican, do you live somewhere with a climate similar to Puerto Rico's, like southern Florida, or are you in Minnesota?)
2. How did your parents approach their health when you were young? Were they fitness fanatics or couch potatoes? Consider the way you ate as a kid. Was yours a no-sugar-allowed household or was it PopTarts and Bagel Bites all the time?
3. Are there diseases that run in your family like diabetes, heart disease, or obesity? What about allergies?
4. Describe where you live now. What's the climate like? Is it urban or rural? How is the air quality?
5. Think about your average day. What's your job like? Your family life? Do you have stressful days but healthy ways of relaxing and unwinding, or do you feel as if you can never get off the stress roller coaster?
6. What is your mom's skin like? What about your

grandmothers' skin? What do you know about their skin-care routines?

7. Think honestly and with as little judgment as you can about your body. (Easier to say than to do, I know, but try your best.) If you didn't feel pressure to look a certain way, if there were no *Sports Illustrated* swimsuit issues or Beyoncé videos, could you be happy and comfortable with the way it actually feels to have your body? Meaning, your weight, your strength, your energy, your flexibility—are they about right, or does something seem off? (You'll need to take some time with this question, it's a tough one.)

YOUR BACKGROUND

The first step in planning how you can have better health and better skin is to understand where you came from—your background. Ethnicity, geography, and your childhood are all crucial in shaping how your health manifests today. Think about the ways that your genetic past and your actual present might or might not match. Does your family tree have narrow roots, or do they spread all over? Did your parents move across the planet, and then, as soon as you grew up, did you move again?

Any session with a new client begins with these questions. When you go to the doctor he or she takes an extensive history, right? Well, so do I. That's because your history and background affect everything about you. You don't need to become a geneticist, just do a little bit of digging and ask a few questions. Did your mom have insane breakouts at your age? Were your ancestors born in the tropics and now you're living in North Dakota? Is every single woman in your family super-curvy, including you? Here are some principles you can expect to find true based on your background:

You have a body type . . . and it's probably very similar to that of someone else in your family. You can shift it a bit, but you will not change its structure. When you think about your body, does it match what you generally see in your family, or are you an outlier? What are your family's eating and exercise habits today, and are yours similar or different? How physically active were you growing up? Just thinking through these kinds of questions probably reveals a few glimmers of insight into why you have an easy time—or a tough one—maintaining the body you want.

My sister is a tiny, tiny human. She has been that way her whole life. She was a size 0 well into her twenties. I was like her until I was about . . . ten years old. I hit puberty and got super-curvy. I used to be really mean to her and say things like, "Just wait till you turn my age, it's gonna happen to you, too!" But I was wrong. That day never came. We have completely different bodies. I am curvy, with a tendency to bulk up when I lift weights. She can eat and do whatever she wants and continues to look like a tiny ballerina. If you see photos of my mom at her age, you would mistake them for twins. If you see my dad at my age, the same is true for us. My sister and I are never going to swap places, no matter how much my thirteen-year-old self wants us to. The same is true for you.

People slightly shift their body shapes by working really, really hard for years and years and being insanely diligent about their eating. The better thing to do is to accept your shape. That doesn't mean to give in to your cravings, it means to pursue a version of health that is appropriate to your body type. If you don't, you will waste a lot of time yearning for something that simply isn't going to happen. Be the healthiest version of you possible, but if you're rocking Kardashian curves, you have no business aspiring to look like Kate Moss. You will end up with unhealthy habits and an unhappy life. And vice versa. I honestly think it can be harder for a naturally tiny person to understand this point because our society has done such a thorough job linking skinniness with health. That's a big mistake. Body weight is generally not an indication of health, and both unhealthy and healthy come in any size.

Your ancestry matters. A million and one dietary theories have been built on this concept. The Paleo Diet encourages you to eat like your ancestors. The Blood Type Diet claims your blood type influences how your body processes foods. Ayurveda is a holistic system of medicine that suggests even your moods and disposition are influenced by your ancestry. While the jury is still out on just how much of an impact our ancestry has on our current health, it certainly is a factor.

According to biologist Rob Dunn, the author of *The Wild Life of Our Bodies*, "If you want to eat what your body 'evolved to eat' you need to eat something different depending on who your recent ancestors were."[5] It makes sense: different people adapted to eat the foods that were available to them, and they passed those adaptations down to later generations.

For example, if your ancestors are Asian, African, Indian, or Hispanic, you are more likely to be lactose intolerant than if they're European. It doesn't matter where you live now or whether you are experiencing symptoms—chances are, you are not processing dairy as easily as someone of Caucasian descent. Similarly, the blood of some Japanese immigrants living in the United States shows extremely high levels of cholesterol compared with other immigrant groups, indicating that the Japanese have a harder time processing American foods than do other immigrant groups (and that where you came from affects how you digest foods in new locations).[6] Different ethnicities have varying amounts of the enzyme needed for processing alcohol and therefore feel its effects very differently. There is a whole world in your ancestry, so it's extremely helpful to learn a little about it. It'll often lead to a couple of tweaks that will make you feel better quickly.

So much in common, head to toe...

LIVED IN NEBRASKA

FINE HAIR

FRECKLES, ROSEY CHEEKS, BLUSHES VERY EASILY

LIVES IN NEW ORLEANS

FAVE FOOD: CORN ON THE COB

FULL CHEST
CURVY HIPS

I ♥ NOLA

ALMOND MILK

FAVE FOOD: CORN ON THE COB

CHURNED BUTTER

BRITTLE NAILS THAT GROW SLOW

AVOIDS DAIRY

MILKED COWS

SMALL FEET, MODEST HEIGHT

YOUR GREAT GRANDMA

YOU

It takes time to change. Many of my clients have vastly different lifestyles as adults than they had when they were growing up. Maybe they've moved far from home or they no longer play a sport, or maybe they grew up in a meat-and-potatoes household and now they're vegan. All of these changes are part of our health backgrounds and factor into the overall picture of our current well-being.

It's important to be patient with your body and to understand that it takes a huge amount of time to adjust to drastic changes. You know those bowls of Froot Loops you ate every single morning until you graduated from college? Sadly, in a way, they're still inside you. You can't eat one salad and then be outraged that your skin isn't immediately better.

Physical activity is another important area to consider. So many of us played sports or took classes when we were younger and moved our bodies regularly, all the time. For me, it was dance. I danced every single day after school and for hours on the weekends. During summers, we'd sometimes have eight-hour rehearsals. And now when I'm busy or lazy, I get frustrated that I can't feel as good by just running twenty minutes a day. But of course I can't. It's not what my body thinks of as normal based on my history.

Retraining your body to expect something new takes time. When you move from a warm place to a cold one, you will probably want to wear five sweaters every winter for the first few years. Meanwhile, your Canadian friends will be able to wear T-shirts when they come to visit you. The same concept applies to your metabolism and your skin. Every time you move to a new climate (or if you travel a lot), or make changes in your diet or your routine, remember this.

Be gentle with your skin and your body as they get comfortable in your new surroundings.

You have a skin type, but not in the way you think. Every day, customers worried about their skin issues send e-mails to my company. And they almost always start out in the same way: "I have combination skin. My T-zone is really oily, but I'm dry everywhere else, and I break out on my chin and forehead. But if I use any products, then I peel and crack like a zombie." What these people think they're doing is describing their skin type. In other words, they believe this is what their skin is *prone to*, no matter what they do.

But terms like "combination skin" and "T-zone" are purely marketing hype. Porcelain skin—that's a skin type. Very dark skin. Skin that always looks sun-kissed. Freckles. Being redheaded. Albino. Those are all skin types. Oily skin, dry skin, blemishes—those are all symptoms. They may be temporary or long-term symptoms, but they are symptoms with solutions.

Honestly, skin type—your actual skin type—doesn't amount to much as far as products go. It does influence how sun exposure affects you. It does influence whether you are prone to developing wrinkles at a younger age. But the products themselves don't really matter; the way you use them matters. African skin is less prone to sunburn but needs more moisture. Fair skin is very quick to burn in the sun and will generally be more sensitive to overcleansing. Mediterranean skin rests somewhere in the middle and should really be what we call "combination" skin. It needs regular moisture and regular cleansing. And, in America, at least, most of us are at least some mixture of all of the above, so our routines really do have to be completely individualized.

Just like your body type, you're not going to change your skin's natural appearance with a product or anything else . . . and you shouldn't try to. You will just have a slightly different routine to manage the symptoms that arise from your background, lifestyle, and diet.

LIFESTYLE

Now that we've gotten through your health past, let's move on to your present. Where you live, where you work, what your family life is like. Do you love your job or hate it? Do you work an insane number of hours? Do you have children? Do you exercise a little, a lot, or not at all? Do you take lots of supplements? Are you on medications? Birth control? Do you smoke cigarettes? Every little detail about your life affects you and your skin. Sometimes I marvel at how much our bodies and skin are actually handling (I know, I'm weird).

Nurture Your Nature

Scientists are learning more every day about the ways in which our lifestyle choices influence our DNA. Epigenetics, an emerging field of genetic research, focuses exclusively on how environmental and lifestyle factors affect the expression of our genetic code. And what these scientists are learning—that the quality of the food we eat and the ways we live our lives factor into whether or not we develop diseases—is amazing. For example, let's say you were born with genes that elevate your risk for heart disease or cancer. Just because you have the genetic disposition to develop these illnesses doesn't mean you'll definitely become sick. The gene could be triggered or not triggered depending on other factors that affect cell health. What you do, where you live, and what you eat matters.

Even more interesting is the notion that you might "turn on" a gene through your lifestyle and then pass it on to your children and even grandchildren. In one study, the grandchildren of men who went through food shortages between the ages of nine and twelve had higher-than-average life spans, while the grandchildren of men who had plenty to eat during those years had life spans that were drastically shortened by heart disease and diabetes.[7] Fascinating! The possibilities for this research (and for the impact of your lifestyle on your future) are huge.

Where You Live

Let's start with your actual physical environment. You already know that your health can be affected by big geographical moves, like when your parents or grandparents left their homeland to start a family in an all-new culture and climate, but where you live now, regardless of your background, also has a huge impact on your body and your skin.

If you live in an urban area, pollution and poor air quality can wreak havoc on your skin by causing inflammation and premature aging. When you live in a big city, your skin is constantly in overdrive trying to fight the elements. Urban areas tend to have very low rates of skin cancer (probably because those who live in urban areas usually get way less sun exposure and have better access to doctors) but high rates of basically every other skin-related ailment.

On the other hand, growing up in a rural area can have amazing benefits for your body's immune system because, as a baby, you get exposed to more kinds of bacteria (think dirt, animals, pollen, plants, etc.). Your body develops antibodies in response to contact with these various microbes that help to boost your immune system for the rest of your life. Unfortunately, though, you can't just pick up one of these supercharged, country immune systems later in life. City dwellers who move to rural places as adults may experience rashes and allergic reactions.

Dry climates tend to dry out your skin (I know, big surprise), especially when the humidity is lower than 30 percent. And because dry climates tend to make your skin crack and peel—making the skin's barrier function weaker—you also become more susceptible to allergens. For example, eczema, psoriasis, and dermatitis tend to flare up more easily in these climates. In humid places, skin is able to retain more of its natural moisture, though sometimes this can result in an overproduction of the oils that leave skin shiny and clog pores. High humidity can also increase the risk of many bacterial and fungal infections that thrive in moist environments. And you will obviously sweat more, which, if you don't take proper care of your skin, can also clog your pores.

Hot climates tend to induce irritating skin conditions like rashes and itchiness, and to also have more intense, direct sun; people who live in hot areas have a higher risk of sunburn. Cold temperatures are generally also very dry, so you are dealing with double the effects. Cold wind results in skin chapping and windburn, and if you use harsh soaps and detergents, you will experience significantly more sensitivity and irritation in the cold. And finally, if you're living at a high altitude, you're dealing with a very combative environment. The sun is strong, the cold is strong, and the wind is strong. Your skin will be more susceptible to burning, chapping, and sensitivity.

Where You Work

Isn't it interesting that any discussion about how work affects health is really a discussion about stress? I so wish it wasn't like that! Stress can exacerbate acute skin conditions such as hives, psoriasis, and rosacea. Nerve endings in your skin relate emotional responses from your brain into actual, physical effects in the skin. For example, sudden fear causes blood to withdraw from the skin as a protective mechanism so that, if you're being attacked by a bear, let's say, you don't bleed as much. That's why your skin feels cold and clammy when you get scared. Crazy, right? But really it isn't surprising when you consider how much of human emotional life plays out physiologically in our skin: blushing from embarrassment, turning red from anger, becoming pale from grief.

So it should also make sense that stress has real effects on your skin. For example, when you are tense, your body releases stress hormones that increase oil production and make you more prone to breakouts. And you've maybe heard of cortisol, another stress hormone that triggers an elevation in blood sugar, damages collagen and elastin, and creates what we call worry lines and wrinkles. During stress, there is also an unhealthy increase in blood flow that causes your capillaries to expand and turns your skin red in the not-cute way.

Feeling unfulfilled has a subtler effect on your health, but it can be equally devastating. The problem with being unhappy with your life isn't just that it usually comes with an increase in those stress hormones; it also makes you significantly less likely to take care of yourself. You know the days when you are just not having it? The days when all you want to do is sit on the couch with a bag of chips and catch up with the *Housewives* and the newest *Bachelor*? Those are not really the days when you get a nice workout, eat a healthy dinner, and whip up a nourishing DIY skin-care treatment. If you are in a rut, or if you hate your job, your home, or another aspect of your life, it can create the prolonged effect of feeling too down to do anything about it. People who have gorgeous skin usually don't hate their lives, and they spend more time taking care of themselves.

I'd say about three out of four of the clients who come to me feeling devastated about their skin work at jobs they can't stand. They feel unfulfilled, unappreciated, uncreative, and—surprise, surprise—ugly. As a person who quit a good, full-time job in the middle of the Great Recession and started a company in her apartment's kitchen, I always want to shake these beautiful, smart, talented women, and say, "Leave that job! Be brave, I promise it'll all be fine." But I know that everybody's circumstances are different, and it's not always that easy.

Your Stress Level

The good news is that, whether or not you make a total life change, combating stress and lack of fulfillment is much easier than you think and equally as powerful. When you reduce stress, you prevent your body from releasing the hormones and chemicals that cause inflammation. One way to do this is by meditating regularly. I know you've heard it before, but it's really true: meditation reduces stress and increases happiness within one twenty-minute session, even if you've never done it before.[8] And if you're not into meditation, consider that your view of stress is actually part of what makes you stressed! In a recent study of 30,000 people, it was discovered that people who perceived stress as bad for their health were significantly more negatively impacted by it than those who perceived it as a normal part of life.[9] So stop stressing about your stress because it only produces more stress!

For the parts of your life that feel gross—an unfulfilling job, lazy habits, a bad relationship, toxic friendships—try setting what are called "implementation intentions."[10] An implementation intention is the conscious declaration (don't worry, you can say it silently in your head) to actually take the steps that are needed to make a big life change. So if you want to leave your soul-crushing job, but you feel that you can't just up and quit, decide, "I'm going to quit my job," and you'll find ways to make it possible. It can be that simple.

One way to begin incorporating healthier habits into your life is to start super-small. Dr. B. J. Fogg, a psychologist at Stanford University, developed a theory of behavior change that is the foundation for his popular method of incorporating "tiny habits"[11]—sometimes as tiny as flossing one tooth, getting into a push-up position, or opening a book. So if you wish you were meditating for twenty minutes a day, decide that you're just going to make a habit of closing your eyes and breathing for one minute. Next, place that tiny habit after some other habit you already have. Maybe you'll do your one-minute session after you brush your teeth in the morning. Doesn't it sound much easier to make a habit of meditating for *one* minute at a set time every day rather than for twenty?

It is. And before you know it, the habit will naturally happen. If you want to stop sitting at your desk so much at work, just make the decision to stand up and sit back down after every task you finish, and then make this a habit. Don't forget to be proud of yourself for doing it. According to Dr. Fogg, that's important, too!

So close your eyes, take a deep breath, and tell the stress to back off. Your skin will get better! But if that sounds too tough for now, at least apply a DIY mask while stalking your ex on Facebook. Cool?

Your Level of Physical Activity

Remember how stress can cause an unhealthy increase in blood flow? Well, exercise causes the kind of increased blood flow that is great for your skin. Exercise helps bring oxygen and nutrients to your skin cells and helps you eliminate waste (through sweat).

One study on the benefits of exercise on skin had sedentary people over the age of sixty-five begin a light workout regimen: two days a week of thirty minutes of moderate cardio, no heavy weights or anything hard-core, just jogging and cycling.[12] Within three months they had regained skin qualities normally seen in people in their twenties and thirties. The stratum corneum, which is the visible layer of the skin, tends to get thick and saggy with age, and the dermis layer tends to become thinner. But the participants in this study saw the stratum corneum thin and become firmer and the dermis layer thicken. That, ladies and gentlemen, means exercise is the only real anti-ager. Too bad it doesn't get its own slick packaging and marketing team.

On the flip side, a sedentary life will age your skin. I find the recently popularized motto "Sitting is the new smoking" to be incredibly motivating. It came about because of a study that showed that sitting for too many hours a day was as bad for your long-term health as smoking. If that's not a reason to get up and move, I don't know what is. Working out also lowers cortisol levels (in other words, it combats stress) and therefore helps to balance the amount of sebum your skin produces. And in some studies, exercise has been shown to be as effective as antidepressants on mental health.[13] So . . . exercise has a physical impact that improves your skin, and it also improves your mood, which prompts you to take better care of your skin. Not to overdo it here, but exercise is practically a cure-all for your skin. That magic elixir we've all been looking for is actually a dumbbell.

If you are having trouble motivating yourself to exercise, two tricks that have worked well for my clients are finding a fun activity and taking along a workout buddy. Do not make yourself do a workout that you hate. You won't keep doing it, and you won't get much benefit from it when you do exercise. Do not feel pressured by the latest fitness trend: there is no one right way to work out. There just isn't. Some people love yoga; others love CrossFit. One is not a better or healthier option than the other. While all of us couch potatoes sit around and argue about which form of exercise is technically superior, those who are actually out there doing it are living the best life ever, with perfect bottoms and glowing skin. The point is that they have found workouts that work for them. They love it, and you should love what you're doing, too.

If you don't love any workout at all, then drag someone along with you. I promise you the number one reason a good personal trainer is effective is because he or she is there to keep you company and hold you accountable. A buddy does the same thing. Next time you have a happy-hour girlfriend date, go to yoga first. Or if you are meeting for brunch, take a spin class before. Together. Even that hot/awful/chipper/insane teacher will be easier to deal with if your friend is there suffering through the class with you.

The only downside to lots of exercise is that you need to be careful about cleaning your skin. Dirty pores will lead to breakouts, and sweating a lot can also make your skin itchy and sensitive. This doesn't mean you need to be using harsh detergent cleansers—especially since they will strip your skin of its natural protective bacteria. But it does mean you'll need to be more diligent about gently cleansing.

Your Overall Health

When we look at the impact of medical conditions on your health and your skin, things can get a little tricky, because we're really talking about two related issues: the condition itself plus the impact of any medication you might be taking to treat it. Very generally, medical conditions will often be accompanied by a weakened immune system, causing you to have more sensitive skin. If your body is compromised, your skin cells will be as well. Plus, when you are sick, your immune system has more important things to worry about than how glowing and happy your skin looks, so it will prioritize healing the struggling organ. Autoimmune diseases, especially, can wreak serious havoc on skin, bringing with them all sorts of rashes, bumps, redness, and sores that are slow to heal on their own.

All of this means that you must be very gentle and careful with your skin while dealing with a serious medical condition.

In essence, you are stepping in to do the work that your body can't. So you may need to be especially mindful of cuts and scrapes, washing them well—sometimes with a stronger soap than I might otherwise recommend. Or, if you find that your skin tears more easily, you may want to skip any kind of abrasive exfoliation.

In addition, most medications have some less-than-desirable side effects. Antibiotics are one example. By being tough on the harmful bacteria, they are also tough on the rest of the bacteria in your body, especially those that live in your gut. Healthy gut bacteria (the microbes that live in your intestinal lining and play a role in everything from digestion to your immune health) are essential to good skin, and every time you take a course of antibiotics, you are wiping them out completely. If you are undergoing or have gone through chemotherapy or radiation, your skin will also suffer. Both treatments slow down the production of fresh skin cells, which will lead to dryness, itchiness, skin that looks aged, a sensitivity to light (photosensitivity), and sometimes hyperpigmentation. Clients going through cancer treatments will find a lot of relief by adding a heavy-duty moisturizer to their routine. Try something with a high percentage of nourishing, gentle cocoa butter or shea butter.

Another common medication, birth control, can cause a form of hyperpigmentation known as malasma, characterized by dark patches that usually appear on the face after spending time in the sun. Birth control can help prevent breakouts by stunting hormones that are responsible for producing excess oil, but that doesn't mean you shouldn't take really good care of your skin even while on birth control. Its skin-clearing effects are the result of a temporary shift in your hormones.

Once you stop taking it, your skin will go back to normal. You want to be happy with what it looks like.

It's important to note that even medications that are meant to help your skin can have unintended consequences. Most commonly, both topical and ingested meds can make your skin insanely dry, chapped, and tender. Many people cannot and should not exfoliate while on acne medication. Topical steroids, which are used to treat many skin conditions, will actually thin and weaken your skin over time. Most acne medication will make you photosensitive. I'm sure you can guess that I am not a fan of taking skin-care medications except in absolute worst-case scenarios. Especially because with or without the side effects, you are treating your symptoms and not correcting the root causes.

The Products You Use

When was the last time you changed your skin-care routine? Have you been using the same line of products for years, or did you recently start something new? Do you change things up every time you run out of a product (or even before)? All three of these behaviors can lead to bad skin for different reasons. Here is what I've found to be generally true for the three categories:

Same routine since you were sixteen. This is usually fine until your late twenties to early thirties. Around this time, most clients who fall into this category start to reject their products. You have to keep in mind that, as you get older, your skin changes. Plus, your entire life is (hopefully) much different than it was in high school. Don't freak out, you're not "old," but you are officially in the "mommy" phase of the skin age spectrum, which I refer to as baby, teen, mommy, grandmommy. It's time to use different products than a teenager uses, Mommy.

You recently switched. So a super-peppy salesgirl talked you into buying a whole new line of products when you were at the department store, but nothing is getting better and the new products don't seem to be working? Stop using them! What's that, you say? The peppy salesgirl told you that you just need time to adjust to the products? She was wrong— this is completely and totally false. Your skin should not get worse before it gets better. Breaking out when you detox is one thing, but breaking out from the products you're using is another. If a new product works for your skin, it should get better almost immediately. You might need two to three days for your pores to clear out some gunk, but beyond that, everything should be amazing. If you've been using a new product for a week and you don't love the results, then it's not for you. And, seriously, if you are in actual physical pain from using a product, *stop now.* Go get a refund from the peppy salesgirl.

You love to change it up. Generally people who frequently change up their skin-care routines have pretty good skin. It's like eating the full rainbow of fruits and vegetables to get a variety of vitamins and minerals—it's nice to give your skin different nutrients, too. But just like with your diet, it's important to have those tried-and-true staples that you always come back to—and it's important to pay attention to changes when you try new things. Too much variety can be overwhelming for your skin. If you are a frequent product swapper and you're having skin problems, then it becomes almost impossible to know what's causing the problem. You may be sensitive to one ingredient that appears in all of the products, or you may be having a reaction to one ingredient that appears in only one of the products. You need to simplify to get clear on what's working and what's not, what's there for fun and what you should toss or skip next time.

What You Believe

This last topic tends to get overlooked in wellness books. Even holistic nutritionists like me fall into the trap of sometimes considering only the facts of our clients' physical health when making our recommendations. But it's important to remember that there can be moral and ethical dimensions to lifestyle choices and that these have real effects on health. For instance, I've had several vegan clients who came to me with chronic skin conditions and some fairly serious health concerns, and it was my determination that these clients—not all vegans, mind you, but these particular ones—were eating the wrong foods for their bodies. I believed that their symptoms would improve if they added healthy animal fats like organic cage-free eggs, fish, and grass-fed butter to their diets, but these clients decided that they would rather not eat animal products, even if doing so might alleviate some of their health problems. The same is often true for people with certain religious traditions. For those of us who don't feel the same kinds of ethical restrictions, it's easy to see some eating styles as simply dietary choices. But often they're better treated as hard facts of a person's lifestyle and, as such, something that must be worked with rather than against.

WHAT YOU EAT

Maybe you thought we'd already covered everything that could possibly factor into your everyday health? Not even close. Your diet gets its own section and is going to be a whole lot of what this book is about. That's because it makes up probably 95 percent of what I discuss with my clients.

Let me say, as clearly as I can, *your diet is the most essential tool you have to getting great skin.* You cannot eat crap and have clear skin. Period. You could ignore everything else in this book and just cut out sugar or drink more water, and your skin would get better. But the problem these days is that almost all of us are putting too much stock in what we're being told to eat by people who don't know us, and we're not listening enough to what our bodies really need. We are all individuals. In the same way that all of the factors in your background and lifestyle affect your overall health, they also affect how you should be eating. Your diet changes throughout your life, and it is greatly impacted by your state of mind.

So we're also going to spend some time learning how to listen to your own body tell you how it wants you to eat. I know wellness authors love to say things like that but then it turns out they're really just trying to get you to go on their diet. I'm going to teach you how to find your own diet. And by diet I don't mean *limitation*, I mean *way of eating*. A general way of eating that you know is right for you and that makes you feel good, makes your skin glow, and, above all, allows you to feel freedom—not restriction—when it comes to food.

The reason I don't ascribe to the one-diet-for-everyone approach is because I have seen people experience completely different results with different diets. Almost everyone who comes to me is already eating in a way they were told to eat, a way that they believe is healthy for everyone. But it's not working for *them*. So while we're not going to spend any time talking about a high-sugar, high-salt diet being right for you (sorry), we are going to spend a lot of time talking about the best categories of foods for your skin and the ways to figure out which foods you should start to incorporate more of and which you might want to skip. It's going to be a lot easier than you think, and you'll be amazed by the impact on your skin and your overall health.

As a side note, supplements are not the answer to your dietary woes. You do not need to supplement vitamins and minerals, you need to eat better. The supplement industry is as big and as dirty as the personal-care industry (more on that soon). Sometimes supplements are necessary, and in Chapter 4 I'll share some of my favorites, but most of the time supplements should be used only when your immune system is struggling. Even then, they are a temporary solution. You should think of every vegetable, fruit, whole grain, protein, and fat as a supplement. You can get every nutrient you need through your food; you just have to actually *consume* the right things. And contrary to your worst fears, carbs and fat are good for you, too. Clear skin comes from good, healthy, wholesome food.

It does not, on the other hand, come from eating lots of sugar, salt, and processed foods. In fact, these are the foods that are giving you sad, sucky skin. It's actually a fairly obvious connection: when you are eating foods that are depleted of vitamins and minerals, you aren't getting vitamins and minerals. Since these nutrients are essential to good skin, you will not have it without them. Sounds basic, but it's a connection a lot of us haven't really made yet. So while I really do believe nutrition and health are very personal, we are going to talk about some of the simple facts, including that some foods are bad for you, some are great for you, and the rest are somewhere in the middle. Our journey together is largely going to be about cutting out some of the bad, adding lots of the good, and unlocking your own perfect diet.

WHEN WE WERE IN kindergarten, our teachers told us that everyone is like a snowflake—no two people are alike. We've known our whole lives that our personalities and likes and dislikes are unique to us as individuals—but we rarely make that same connection about our own, individual biology. Because we are each made up of a different mix of genetic and lifestyle factors, no two of our bodies work in exactly the same way—which is why your friend may use one skin-care product with great success, but that same product makes you break out; or why another friend can eat dairy and have clear skin, but if you have one bite of ice cream, it's all over. No two people are completely alike, and no two will have exactly the same skin; therefore, no two people should be doing exactly the same things for their skin. Your skin-care regimen should be individual and personalized.

There are a million different tiny details that make up who you are. Which means you shouldn't be eating exactly the same as someone else, working out exactly the same as someone else, or treating your skin exactly the same as someone else. And while you cannot escape your background, you also don't have to let it control you. I've had clients who prefer to keep dairy in their diets even if they find that it makes them break out once in a while. I've had vegan clients who struggle with their energy levels or with keeping weight on, so they make up for it by snacking. I use these examples to say that you are going to use the tools in this book to come up with *your own routine*, whether or not it has some compromises in it. The bottom line is that it's important to remember that all of the factors above are at play in your life, at all times.

Don't worry, you're going to see how this all fits together really soon.

CHAPTER 3

YOUR BODY NEEDS YOU

Now it's time we get to the nitty-gritty and answer the million-dollar question that is probably what inspired you to pick up this book in the first place: Where are your skin problems coming from? Fair warning, you may not like some of the answers. But trust me, there's a light at the end of the tunnel. Just stick with me, friend, we'll get there; and on the other side is beautiful, glowing skin.

THE BEAUTY ENEMIES

Common skin issues generally arise from the same, systemic cause: normal bodily functions gone haywire. One of the things that regulates those bodily functions? Hormones.

Hormones regulate practically everything that makes us human: digestion, breathing, sleep, sex, reproduction. And while we generally do tend to overblame our hormones as the culprit for things like our slow metabolism and mood swings, they really are a large part of why our skin freaks out.

Hormonal changes during puberty, menstruation, and menopause all impact the skin. Estrogen affects skin thickness, firmness, and moisture levels, and it has anti-inflammatory properties, which is why, when estrogen drops off during menopause, skin tends to become flushed, dry, and less elastic. Testosterone is involved in sebum production, which can lead to acne, so that's why so many of us get acne during puberty and when we're on our periods—two times when testosterone levels are elevated.

But hormones affect everyone a little bit differently. So your skin problems aren't necessarily occurring because your hormones are out of whack; you might have totally normal hormone levels that your body has a different response to than another woman's body might. That's why every woman's period affects her differently and why some women never, ever break out, no matter what stage of life they're in. If you've never had an issue with acne, that means your body has always been okay with your changing hormone levels. If you have, then you are sensitive to the changes. Don't worry, most of us are.

You want to know the best way to keep your hormones balanced? With your diet. It seems like a no-brainer, but it's actually the last thing most of my clients think of when it comes to hormone regulation. One of the major culprits in hormonal imbalance is fat intake. A diet too light in fruits and vegetables and too heavy in processed and industrialized foods (like factory-farmed meat and pasteurized dairy) can definitely create a hormonal imbalance. But our obsession with a low-fat diet has also really messed up our hormones. Healthy fats—like coconut oil, avocado, wild-harvested cold-water fish, olive oil, and even organic grass-fed butter—are crucial to keeping hormone levels healthy. I've had a few clients who were so afraid of eating fat that they actually no longer got their periods at all. And these were women in their twenties and thirties. Fat will not make you fat—but not eating enough of it could make you break out and even develop more serious health issues.

Another big beauty enemy is inflammation. In fact, it's not just a beauty enemy, it is a *public enemy*. More and more, doctors and researchers are finding that inflammation is actually the root cause of the majority of our health problems these days, including many deadly diseases. So let's take a quick minute to talk about what inflammation actually is.

Your body produces an inflammatory response to protect and heal itself. Think of bumping your shin on the coffee table. The worst, right?! Well, the swollen red bump that forms afterward is actually good for you. It's the result of your body rushing blood and fluid to the area to repair any damage that's been caused. The same is true for a fever, which is another kind of inflammatory response. During a fever, your whole body is trying to fight off an invader, whatever bacteria or virus is making you sick. A pimple is another inflammatory response triggered by the presence of foreign bacteria.

The problem is not really that your body is having an inflamed response; it's how often that response happens and how long it lasts. There's a difference between *acute* inflammation, which is a specific, brief episode, like what happens when you bang your shin on the table, and *chronic* inflammation, which is implicated in conditions like arthritis, eczema, psoriasis, celiac disease, allergies, and many, many others. In chronic inflammation, something triggers the body's immune response even though there is no external invader, no bacteria or virus, to attack. As a result, healthy cells suffer. It's a little bit like if you had a really loyal—but vicious—guard dog, and you loved having guests over. While he's the best dog ever if there are robbers at your door, when your friends come over, he's kind of a problem. Inflammation is an overdrive response to an alerted body. It's a stress response.

And these days, most of us are in this stress response all the time. Our modern lifestyles are full of stressors, from environmental pollution to credit card debt to Twitter drama. But our diets are also big sources of chronic inflammation. The problem foods are no surprise: processed sugars, trans fats, too much meat, and refined grains. So even if you aren't suffering from a disease, a diet full of these kinds of foods will keep you chronically inflamed just as if you were, and when you are inflamed all the time, your skin suffers the consequences.

Glycation—also a normal bodily process that can go wrong—is another culprit in skin damage and aging. Glycation occurs when your body tries to digest and process an influx of sugar, and fat or protein molecules bond to the sugar molecules without an enzyme present to control the reaction. That little enzyme is crucial. With the enzyme, a process called glycosylation takes place, which is good and normal and essential to healthy cellular function. Without it, you get glycation, which produces a kind of crazy, Frankenstein sugar-protein substance called an advanced glycation end product or an AGE (an appropriate name considering the fact that AGEs destroy youthful, glowing skin).

Here's why AGEs are bad: your body doesn't know what to do with them. Because they're sugars that haven't been metabolized correctly, your body looks at them as foreign substances and produces antibodies to attack them. Meaning, it treats the AGE as if it's an infection. And we now know what happens when you get an infection: your body produces an inflammatory response. In skin, this inflammation leads to premature wrinkling and sagging, but the effects of AGEs have been linked to more serious health consequences, too, such as diabetes, Alzheimer's, and heart disease. AGEs are at the root of how inflammation messes up your skin.

And AGEs aren't only produced within the body, they're also in foods—I probably don't even need to tell you which ones, but basically if it's sugary, processed, fried, or too meaty, there's a good chance it contains AGEs. Foods cooked at high temperatures—especially animal protein (think: burgers on the grill, fried chicken)—are especially prone to developing AGE molecules. Shocked? Neither am I. Sad about it? Me, too.

Last but definitely not least, free radicals (created by yet another normal bodily process) are a huge beauty enemy. Free radicals are just molecules with a single, unpaired electron—most molecules have two. They're created when our cells take in and use oxygen, and they are a normal, inevitable part of being alive. They're not even all bad: when everything is working right, free radicals allow your cells to communicate with one another and help important reactions in our body take place, and they are a normal by-product of the aging process.

One of the reasons the beauty industry is so obsessed with anti-aging products is because, like the rest of the body, the skin does naturally weaken and become deficient with age. It actually is true that the processes associated with aging in the skin can happen fast or slow depending on how well our bodies deal with free radicals. The problem is that when there are too many free radicals present in the body, they can do some major damage. Because they have that unpaired electron, they're always hunting for other molecules to react with. They're like the north pole of a magnet looking for a south pole to latch onto. That often means they end up latching onto DNA or attacking cell membranes and wreaking havoc. Free radicals have been linked to cell damage and cell death, leading not just to the thinness and looseness of aging skin, but also to severe health concerns like stroke, heart disease, even cancer. So unchecked free radicals are serious business—not just for the health of our skin but for our overall well-being and longevity.

When we're young and healthy, our bodies have an antioxidant defense system that keeps the production of free radicals in check. Antioxidants react with free radicals and neutralize them, and they also stop them from continuing to cause more damage and more free-radical creation. But as we grow older the production of free radicals naturally overpowers our antioxidant system, and when we eat badly and expose ourselves to environmental and life stresses, that process speeds up.

So your body does synthesize antioxidants and do a lot of the defense work on its own—because it's magical—but mostly you get the strength you need to combat free radicals from your diet. Vitamins E, C, and beta-carotene are three of the most powerful antioxidants, and they are in virtually every healthy food you can imagine: fruits, nuts, leafy green vegetables. And among the many habits and foods that contribute to an increase in free radicals are smoking, drinking alcohol, and the chemical preservatives in food and in gross, industrial skin care.

BIG KIDS KEEP FOOD JOURNALS

Okay, I know what you're thinking. This is the point where all of my clients say some version of the same thing: "OMG, everything I eat causes hormonal imbalance, inflammation, glycation, and free radicals. I give up! Pass the pepperoni pizza." Well, I'll tell you the same thing I tell them when they start to throw this little temper tantrum, and it's really going to bum you out. It's something we all already know is true, deep down. We surround ourselves with people who never mention it and get rid of people who bring it up too much. It's okay, but we're going to have to deal with it now. Are you ready?

You are an adult now.

Ouch, I know. It's taken me about ten years of fighting and complaining before I finally realized I needed to just accept that fact. I cannot tell you how many times I have proclaimed in my adult life that something pertaining to my health isn't fair. It's not fair that I burn in the sun. It's not fair that I can't eat whatever I want without its affecting me. It's not fair that I have to work out; otherwise, I start to hurt in places I didn't know could hurt. It's not fair that I have to take care of my skin and hair and it doesn't just naturally look sexy all the damn time. You know who thinks things aren't fair all the time? Children. I hope it takes you less time than it took me to come to terms with the fact that life isn't about fairness. It's about doing the best you can with what you've been given.

Every client I've ever worked with has some kind of terrible habit that basically stems from an inability to accept this idea. Every single one! Their terrible habits are usually coffee or bacon. Maybe yours is wine or cheese or ice cream. It's all the same. You are, sadly, subject to the consequences of your choices. We all are. There are foods that are good for you and foods that are bad for you. You cannot binge eat without consequences. You cannot treat your skin and your body like crap and expect it to bounce back, no problem. And, yes, you will get wrinkles.

The reason I mapped out the scary culprits of your bad skin—hormones, inflammation, glycation, and free radicals—was to show you how they are all connected. And they are connected by something you can control: food. Bad food is just bad for you. There is no way to get around it. So while we are going to spend time getting to the bottom of what *your* best foods and *your* worst foods are, you'd better believe sugar, fried foods, and processed foods are not on *anyone's* list of best foods. They are beauty enemies no matter who you are, how much you exercise, where you live, or how wonderful your genes are.

In other words, what you eat really matters, and there's no way around it. It's never going to be the case that junk food will make you feel great, and it's very possible that there are actually some foods that you think are awesome that are impairing you. The truth is that nutrition science changes constantly, and much is still shrouded in mystery. Your body's response is incredibly personal and specific to you. That sexy guilt-free super-food powder you drink in your homemade shake every morning with $100 worth of organic ingredients in it? It could be part of your problem. So while there are some foods that, no question, you have to get rid of (there isn't anyone in the universe, ever, for whom deep-fried cheese is a health food), it's also important to find *your very own* problem foods. Until you do that, knowing what's causing your skin issues will always be a guessing game.

And here's how you're going to do it: with a little tool called a **food journal**. Maybe you've heard of this new trendy way of feeling really crappy about how you eat. But it's totally worth the pain, I promise. A food journal really does help you simplify your diet and identify the foods that could be triggering problems, for your skin and otherwise.

A food journal is exactly what it sounds like: a personal diary in which you log what you eat and drink, along with your physical symptoms. Then you either show your journal to a professional to evaluate, or you learn to evaluate it yourself. The accumulated information is enlightening and often a little bit shocking. If you are totally, totally honest with yourself, you'll very quickly spot all sorts of foods you didn't even notice you were eating until you began to write down every morsel that passed your lips.

Recently, food journals have been utilized by health coaches and nutritionists to help people spot allergies and sensitivities. This is extremely important. You may not have full-blown food allergies, but you can have a fairly wide range of foods to which you are sensitive. I've seen lists that included dairy, all grains, eggs, soy, and corn. All in one person! Sensitivities to different foods are at the root of bad skin because they trigger low-level immune responses and, therefore, inflammation. Since they don't cause massive reactions, it's easy to overlook them, which means you keep eating the food. Eventually, the inflammation becomes chronic. Whether or not you can feel it, when you are not properly metabolizing food, you are not properly absorbing nutrients, and, therefore, you are causing more inflammation. Think of it this way: bad nutrition equals inflammation equals skin problems.

On top of this, sometimes overconsumption of a food will

lead to a reaction in your body that is similar to a sensitivity or an allergy, except that it's only temporary. If you suspect you may be having a reaction to a staple in your diet, your naturopathic doctor can order a blood test that will reveal any flare-ups caused by overconsumed foods. I once took the test and discovered I was having a reaction to blueberries, flax-seeds, and strawberries. The three ingredients I was putting in smoothies virtually every day . . . because they're healthy!

You don't need to get a blood test in order get a better sense of your food sensitivities, though. Keeping a detailed food journal should help you spot your own problem foods. Just keep in mind that the point of keeping a food journal is to learn, not to judge. I believe it is extremely important not to journal for longer than two weeks. I don't care what anyone says, unless you are allergic to everything and need to keep close tabs for reactions, food journaling every day is a form of calorie counting (which is why food journals are common in dieting programs). It's an unfortunate side effect of our culture, and for many of us it's almost impossible not to become obsessed once we start writing everything down. I've seen it happen many times. But you're not going to do that. Keep your journal for a bare minimum of three days. A full week will make all of your problems crystal clear, and two weeks will give you time to straighten yourself out. You can always come back to food journaling when you've lost your way or need to readjust some things. But otherwise, in as little as three days, you're going to be blown away by how much you've learned about your eating habits and your body's (and skin's) reactions to the foods you eat.

So here's how you're going to keep your food journal:

For at least three days and at most two weeks, you're

going to write down absolutely everything you ingest—meals, drinks, medicines, supplements, snacks, even those little nibbles that "don't count." You're not showing this to anyone else, so don't go easy on yourself. *Everything* counts. Pay close attention to beverages, including water. They're easy to overlook (and I can almost guarantee you that you're not drinking enough water).

You're also going to keep track of physical symptoms like any headaches, stomachaches, intense hunger pangs, or bloating you may experience. Low energy, bursts of energy, sleepiness, insomnia—these are all things to note in the journal. You should also keep track of emotional shifts, like mood swings. Lastly, you'll add observations about your skin. You might need to check in with your skin a little more closely than you do now, but you need to do so only early in the morning and before bed. Did you wake up with a breakout? Were you super-oily before bed? Did you notice after exfoliating that your skin turned bright red and kind of hurt? Write all of this down.

As a bonus, also add any other tidbits you think are important. Use your intuition. If you think it matters, it probably does. Physical activity, unusual amounts of stress at work, a fight at home, your special time of the month. Write it all down. It's only a few days, and it will change your life. Trust me, even during the food-journaling period, you will feel as if you're holding a mirror up to your entire existence and noticing odd details and indicators you never saw before. Just keeping the journal is a crazy experience. It will nudge you toward the right path because you'll see the problems without my even needing to tell you what they are. But don't worry, I'm also going to tell you what they are.

After you have kept your journal for a few days, you may already be able to tell that you eat a bit more than you'd like and you drink way more wine than you'd realized. That's what most people see first. Take some deep breaths and focus. Remember, we are here to get answers, not to give ourselves stress breakouts. This is about the deeper connections. It's about looking at the journal and getting really clear on *you*. Because there's no point in making changes if they're not the right ones. Keep going and keep writing—don't be afraid.

After you have journaled for the allotted number of days you decided on, it's time to go deep, to analyze your food journal and identify the foods and habits that are causing you problems. Below, you will find two sample food journals and instructions on how to analyze your own. God bless the clients who offered them up for this book, because we all know it's not easy to look at our journals by ourselves, in the privacy of our own homes, let alone share them with the 8 trillion people now reading this international best seller.

Client 1 is a vegetarian-leaning married mother of two who gets eczema on her hands and elbows, and seborrheic dermatitis (itchy, flaky skin on the scalp, in the eyebrows, and around the nostrils). She has been recently experimenting with cooking more vegetarian food for her family; she lives in the suburbs and works from home. She is of European descent, but her family has been in the United States for a few generations.

SATURDAY

7 a.m.: Very large black coffee with three sugars. Bites of kids' leftover organic oatmeal from a packet, organic yogurt, and grapes.

12 p.m. (Lunch out with a business friend): Vegetarian soy chicken Caesar wrap, side of French fries. A few bites of huevos rancheros from friend's

meal. Sweetened iced tea (three sugars) and one glass water.

6 p.m. (Home): Cooked angel hair pasta with cubed halloumi cheese, garlic, olive oil, tomatoes, salt and pepper, and two glasses pinot grigio with dinner. Third glass before bed.

SUNDAY

7 a.m.: Woke up with a headache. Large black coffee, three sugars.

9 a.m. (Breakfast out with family): Cheddar and spinach quiche with a side salad, vinaigrette dressing. Large iced coffee with three sugars, one glass water. Half of one pancake, a few bites scrambled egg (kids' again).

2 p.m.: Four chocolate-covered pretzels, handful of baby carrots, organic string cheese.

4 p.m.: Baked vegan chocolate-chip cookies with kids, ate four.

6 p.m. (Home): Cooked soy sausage with white rice, bottled Teriyaki sauce, and packaged coleslaw, two glasses water. One beer.

MONDAY

7 a.m.: Large black coffee three sugars. Granola bar.

11 a.m.: Peanut butter and jelly sandwich, handful of baby carrots, veggie sticks with hummus.

1 p.m.: Three slices organic deli ham. Large coffee, three sugars.

6 p.m.: Takeout Indian food—potatoes, peas, and cauliflower, spinach in cream sauce, white rice. Two chocolate-chip cookies. Two glasses of water. Super-bloated!

TUESDAY

7 a.m.: Large black coffee, three sugars. Made egg sandwiches on English muffins with American cheese and hot sauce.

11 a.m.: Cup of water. Handful of organic cheese crackers, grapes, and three slices organic deli ham.

1 p.m.: Frozen soy veggie burger on bun and some greens with bottled

vinaigrette. One glass water, one large coffee with three sugars. Chocolate-chip cookie.

7 p.m. (Takeout): Two slices pizza with goat cheese and caramelized onions. One slice plain cheese. Greens with vinaigrette. One beer. Sliced strawberries. Pounding headache, went to bed early.

Client 2 is an omnivore with a very stressful job. Her skin rotates between being really oily and really dry, with constant breakouts. She is single, lives in a big city, travels a lot for work, and was extremely athletic as a kid.

SUNDAY

9 a.m.: Coffee with milk and agave.

1 p.m. (Brunch out): Breakfast burrito with veggies, cheddar, eggs, bacon. Lemonade, two glasses of water. Dessert: split a deluxe milk shake with chocolate brownie pieces with a friend.

9 p.m.: Felt a little gross so no real "dinner" but two glasses of wine, some Oreos.

MONDAY

7 a.m.: Woke up feeling super-sick, nauseous, feverish, had to call out of work. Went back to sleep.

11 a.m. (Leftovers from the fridge): Half a burger (not very hungry). Water.

7 p.m. (Feeling better; hungry and more energetic. Had dinner plans, so went out): One bratwurst, handful of fries. One glass of water, one beer.

TUESDAY

8 a.m.: Iced coffee with half-and-half and one sugar.

11 a.m.: Cup of water.

1 p.m. (No time for lunch at work, grabbed snacks from the break room): Handful of Chex mix, half of a donut, and half of a muffin. Cup of water.

7 p.m. (Still at work for dinner, ordered delivery): Kung Pao chicken and white rice. One Diet Coke.

WEDNESDAY

8 a.m.: Spin class before work.

9 a.m. (At the gym): Smoothie with yogurt, mango, whey powder (that's healthy, right?), soy milk, honey.

10 a.m.: Hot coffee with milk and sugar.

2 p.m. (At work): Half a plate of leftover Chinese food from the night before. Snapple from vending machine.

5 p.m.: Two cups water.

8 p.m. (Home, not that hungry): One bag of microwave popcorn. Two glasses wine.

THURSDAY

Woke up with a breakout and feeling really oily. (Also, it's been really humid outside for a few days.)

8 a.m.: Iced coffee with milk and two sugars.

2 p.m. (Lunch out near work): Three small (I swear) pork tacos on corn tortillas. Snapple.

6 p.m.: Hot yoga class after work with a friend. Tons of water!

8 p.m. (Dinner with friend): One chicken finger, chipotle ravioli (had peppers and cheese and beef and creamy chipotle sauce and was really worth it). Two glasses of red wine. Water.

When You Analyze Your Food Journal, Start Off by Looking for the Red Flags

A red flag can be a not-so-great food that appears over and over in the journal, or it might be any behavior that shows up way more often than you'd like. In both clients' sample journals French fries make an appearance. So does takeout, packaged food, and coffee. (There is almost always a lot of coffee in people's food journals.) There's also a lot of refined food, in the form of either white rice, white bread, alcohol, cookies, granola bars, muffins, and, oh yeah . . . a brownie milkshake. Neither diet includes nearly enough vegetables or fiber.

In your food journal, did you notice you ate pasta six times last week? Did you think you had candy once a week, but it's actually in your journal every single day around lunchtime? Did you skip working out the whole time you were journaling? Do you ever have a dairy-free or sugar-free day? Are you "quitting smoking" by bumming cigarettes from your co-workers? Do vegetables even make an appearance? Does any home-cooked food?

All of these are red flags—and it's normal to have them. You're going to find that you're not quite the eater you think you are, or wish to be. And that's okay, for now. Sometimes it helps to pick a food you see more than once and take a tally to force an awakening in yourself. How many glasses of wine did you drink while you journaled? Six? A dozen? How many pieces of fresh fruit did you eat? One? None? I do an exercise for clients sometimes—count out the number of meals in the journal that include meat, compared with the number that include refined carbs (like white bread or pasta), compared to the number that include fresh fruits and vegetables—and they are never, ever, ever happy about what they see. But it is a very effective eye-opener. Do yourself the ~~punishment~~ favor of trying this exercise. When you see the imbalances between broccoli and burgers, you can't ignore the reality of your food choices anymore. Remember, this part is just about becoming more observant.

Monday, monday...

8:00 AM — Woke up with headache. Bloated.

9:00 AM — this is BREAKFAST, right? GRANDE MOCHA LATTE / PB CARAMEL PROTIEN BAR

11:30 AM — at the meeting — MUST EAT MUFFIN.

1:30 PM — STARVED! HEALTH CHIPS / DIET / MUST STUFF FACE.

2:30 PM — two TINY PB cups — Buffalo Chicken Salad with LITE blue cheese dressing

4:00 PM — leftover meeting muffins have been located... plus more coffee

7:00 PM — A little bit of this, a little bit of that... SALSA

FRO YO — PITA CHIPS — a couple more bites while I relax...

11:30 PM — ZZZ — fell asleep on the couch.

The Second Thing to Look for Is Patterns, Especially When It Comes to Your Symptoms

Look for the headaches or mood swings or breakouts. You'll almost always find a food or product in common with each symptom, and the same is true for positive things like energy, going to the bathroom, and feeling like your belly is flat and happy.

When we looked at my mostly vegetarian client's symptoms, we discovered that dairy and sugar were her biggest culprits. She realized she always felt bloated after meals that contained cream, and she experienced headaches pretty regularly that were directly linked to how much sugar she'd eaten that day. We experimented with only two days of no dairy or sugar, and she felt as if she had better digestion, more energy, and a better general mood. In just two days! Soy was a lesser problem for her, though we did work to cut back her soy consumption because she was hoping to get pregnant again and soy can cause a hormone imbalance. For the omnivore, her physical issues were all linked to the restaurant and processed foods she was eating. We couldn't find a specific ingredient that caused the flare-ups, which is exactly the problem with eating like this. The high number of (processed) ingredients in Oreos, microwaved popcorn, break room snacks at work, and all restaurant food . . . it adds up. When people start cooking a little more and bringing food to work, they slowly but surely feel better, and their skin improves. When I first met this client, she used to call out of work feeling sick at least once a month. She also suffered from constant colds. That all stopped when she cleaned up her diet.

Scan your journal for your own patterns. Do you have headaches if you don't drink coffee by a certain time? Do you wake up the morning after drinking even one glass of alcohol feeling as if you partied at a frat house? Do you feel constipated after you eat out? Did you indulge in a dessert that you don't usually eat and wake up with an itchy rash? Do you get heartburn after drinking carbonated beverages? Did you feel dizzy one day and see you didn't actually drink any water at all? Sometimes the link is actually a combination of things. So it may be that when you eat two foods or types of foods together, you get bloated. It may be that drinking a fresh vegetable juice on its own upsets your stomach, but if you drink a lot of water with it, you feel awesome. I had a client who stopped drinking tea with breakfast and moved it to lunch and felt a million times better.

It is impossible for me to name all of the different combinations of symptoms that are rooted in your diet and habits.

Learning about how your body responds to food is a process of discovery that you have to do for yourself. You have to have an open mind and experiment. Don't be afraid to tweak, and don't jump to extreme conclusions until you make smaller tweaks. One client thought she was sensitive to chickpeas because hummus made her bloated. Then she tried some tahini-free hummus and felt fine. Be patient, and don't give up!

Lastly, Look at the Journals in the Context of Your Background

Remember those questions you answered back in Chapter 2? Here's where you put that information to use. Your sensitivity to certain foods might have a genetic component, or it could be that even though you're not feeling symptoms, thinking about your background might make you notice some red flags that you previously overlooked. For example, do you eat a lot of meat even though your family struggles with high blood pressure and heart disease? Do you eat a ton of sweets but have diabetes in your genes? How is your parents' health in general? Maybe they're super-youthful and healthy, but you feel like crap all the time. If that's the case, you may want to look at your food journal in comparison to how you ate growing up. Maybe your childhood habits were better for you than what you're doing now.

My omnivorous client experimented with working out five times a week instead of two, which is how often she exercised when she first came to me. It was like a whole new world opened up to her. Even though she had little time for exercise, she realized that when she worked out, she felt less stressed, more productive, and more "herself." This is because it *was* more her, since being athletic was a huge part of her past. My vegetarian gal's European parents and grandparents ate a lot of fermented foods. When we started pairing dairy with probiotics, she felt much better. She also didn't eat soy growing up (nor did any of her ancestors), which was another reason I encouraged her to cut back a bit.

Here are a few more common patterns and behaviors I often find when I look at food journals with my clients:

- People love the same comfort foods they ate growing up, and it can be a big weakness. Generally, these foods don't make you feel so great, but you just can't quit them. Also, everyone seems to think they have these foods just "once in a while" when really it's more like every other night. I don't think I have to give you examples, but we'll just say . . . macaroni and cheese.
- Almost always, eating habits are picked up from your family. Whether you like to graze or sit down for big meals, your preference probably dates back to your childhood. Many times when there are health issues, you are resisting what you did while you were growing up. It's sort of like the Freshman Fifteen, but forever.
- As Americans, we all eat a lot of sugar. It pops up all over every single food journal I've ever seen. I don't care if you're trying to be a breatharian, there is sugar all over your food journal. Sometimes the sugar isn't the worst part—it's the guilt and negative associations that come with eating sugar. The clients who indulge in a healthy way, as a special treat, do not usually have physical issues from sugar—yet they feel terrible every time they eat it. If you are eating a piece of your own birthday cake, don't

beat yourself up. But if sugar is in there six times a day, it's most definitely wreaking havoc on your health and skin and should be considered a red flag.

- If you're a vegetarian or a vegan, you're most likely eating too much soy and sugar. This is a problem for most of the vegetarian clients I've worked with, because so many vegetarian restaurants and packaged foods are filled with processed soy and a ton of sugar.
- Meat eaters often eat too much meat. You don't need to have it at every meal, no matter how good it makes you feel. Grass-fed or otherwise. And especially otherwise.
- Pescatarians usually eat too much fish. Given the poor quality of most of the seafood available when you're just grabbing a salad or ordering in dinner, you need to be careful about your consumption of seafood. Eating too much fish these days is just like eating too much factory-farmed meat.
- No one eats enough vegetables. Period.

Obviously, I can't tell you what's right or wrong for you specifically, but what I can tell you with total certainty is that your goal in analyzing your food journal is not to see if you could eat better according to the latest nutritional trend, it's to discover what "better" means for you. A healthful lifestyle and diet will look different from one person to the next. So as you try to make dietary changes to improve your health and the health of your skin—or when you follow any other self-improvement program for that matter—it's important to put suggestions and advice in the context of who you are and what you discovered about yourself in your journal.

Awareness Not Judgment!

One last thing before we move on: I want you to be really aware of self-judgment as you analyze your journal. You're probably doing better than you realize, with a few weaknesses that you didn't know you had. I've seen more journals than I can remember, and most people are surprisingly healthy. I'm always impressed by how hard my clients are trying to be healthy. And then I just have to talk them down from the fifteen cups of coffee a day, or the M&M's jar at work. Or point out something super-specific and seemingly random, like all the flaxseeds and blueberries that are giving them a sensitivity from overconsumption. But the list of self-criticisms I get from the person keeping the journal is always huge, and full of paranoia. Don't do that to yourself! Even if your journal is full of red flags, just by keeping the journal you're taking positive steps toward a healthier way to live. You're doing great!

CLEAN SLATE

Another tool that helps most clients is an elimination diet. An elimination diet is not some complicated detox, and you do not need to throw this book across the room because you were traumatized once by trying to drink disgusting spicy lemonade for ten days. I am talking about a cleanse so easy a baby could do it . . . or already does it? I am talking about picking one or two foods, and taking a twenty- to forty-day break from them.

After analyzing your journal, you've probably noticed that there are some foods that appear every day, or a few times a week. These are likely to be problem foods for you. Chances are, if there is something you really, really love to eat and feel like you could never live without, you could use a break from it. Having problem foods is like being in a crappy relationship. You know you should call it quits, but even after you do, you can't stop thinking about him or her.

Don't freak out. Focus on the fact that the symptom is probably temporary, triggered by overconsumption, and so the break is probably going to be temporary, too. Taking a break from a problem food that you're obsessed with is one of those "if you love it, set it free" things. Most of the time, the symptom will go away and you and your beloved food can get back together and live happily ever after. But if you reintroduce the food and the same symptoms come back, then the breakup needs to be permanent. It's like if you try to get back together with that crappy ex and suddenly think, *What am I doing?!* A clean break is definitely needed. After a while you'll be glad you did it because you'll feel so good! That rash will clear up or you won't get stomachaches every time you eat. Choosing to eliminate something permanently should feel like a relief, not a restriction.

Most of the time you'll find that your culprit foods contain wheat, dairy, meat, sugar, or soy. And for, like, 99.9 percent of you, especially if you're dealing with breakouts, it's cheese. Sorry.

But sometimes it's completely random. People will notice they feel not so great after their daily coffee, or almonds, or fruit. I had one client who was trying to incorporate more raw vegetables into his diet because he'd heard that eating raw was healthier, but he was feeling really lousy. Know what it turned out to be? All the salad dressings in his raw meals were made with cashews. He swapped them out and went right back to feeling like his normal self. We're all different, so you'll have to tune into how you feel to find out which foods are messing you up.

Now that you've analyzed your food journal, identified the problems, and picked a couple of foods to eliminate, be sure to find replacements for the foods you're breaking up with. Don't just cut them out—you will hate your life if you don't swap in something else. So whether it's nondairy milk instead of cow's milk, chicken instead of beef, beans instead of chicken, or dates and prunes instead of gummy bears, you'll need something to make it easier. Then, once you're ready, make the break.

Listen to Your Body, Not Your Mind

Make sure that you are choosing to eliminate a food because your body doesn't want it, not because something you've heard or read has made you question it. It's an important difference. If you are eating a diet that is already low in fat, don't decide to cut out coconut oil because you're convinced fat is the problem. If you are a meat eater who eats quinoa and brown rice, don't just remove them because you read a paleo blog that said grains are evil.

Another iteration of this is when people choose to cut out a food that is easy for them to live without but that makes them feel proud to eliminate. A few clients of mine chose to eliminate coffee—but these were not the caffeine-addicted guzzlers who *should* consider quitting coffee. The point is, if you drink half a cup of coffee a couple of times a week, your elimination diet should not include coffee. Or if you eat one meal out a week, restaurant food probably isn't the issue. You need to really, deeply pay attention to how you feel physically. Sometimes mental reactions to a food are so bad that you experience actual physical symptoms, so in that case I understand deciding to take a break, but remember that this is about getting to the bottom of what foods your body and skin are sensitive to, and your mental reaction may be confusing the issue.

After you've taken a break from your problem foods, try adding them back into your diet one at a time. Don't bring them all back at once or you won't be able to tell what's causing the issue. If one of the foods is indeed a problem for you, a permanent problem, you'll know soon after you eat it. Usually people experience symptoms like indigestion, slightly itchy skin, bloating, or a general run-down feeling almost immediately. It's very similar to an allergic response, but milder.

After you reintroduce the first food, wait three or four days before bringing back the second one. That way any reactions you had to the first food will be reduced and so you won't mistake which food is really causing the problem. If you don't experience any symptoms, you should be able to eat these foods again without any flare-ups. If the problem comes back, then you've found one of your culprit foods. It's your future terrible ex. But in both situations, if you stick to the elimination, your skin will look way better by the end of it all. I swear.

For vegetarians and vegans interested in trying this, please keep in mind that if you don't feel amazing right now, it may be that adding organic, pastured meat to your diet could help you feel better. If you aren't willing to make that change, don't worry, but be prepared to make up for the foods that you eliminate. So if you cut out sugar, add fruit. If you cut out soy, add lots of beans and nuts. And generally, watch your fat intake during this time. Add more coconut products and vegetable oils and avocados. If you are a veggie because you believe it's healthier, but find that you are so sensitive that you cannot digest coconuts, nuts, avocados, and soy, then I beg you to rethink your diet! I have had lots of clients who hated hearing this, but you must be careful. Some people feel amazing by going veggie, and some people feel awful. Don't assume you'll feel great just because you heard that someone else did. If you are veggie for ethical reasons, you will need to pay more attention to the other ways you take care of yourself— things like what skin-care products you use and what supplements you take.

This is true of anyone on a strict diet, for whatever reason. You are trying to fit your unique self into a boxy program. By design, this is a conflict. There will always be places where your biology and background do not totally match the path you've chosen. It's important to pay attention to your body to spot the inconsistencies in your health or your skin. If you are open to making tweaks, that's optimal. If not, be ready to pay more attention and intensify your self-care.

Megan McGrane is a fellow health coach who spent years struggling with her health while no one could give her answers. She is a really great example of someone who didn't fit into a typical eating program, and who made important discoveries though keeping a food journal and doing an elimination diet. I'll let her tell you the story in her own words:

"I have a total of four autoimmune disorders: Raynaud's, celiac, Hashimoto's, and psoriasis. When I was diagnosed with my third one, I was floored. I was a kale-eating, green-juicing, almost-vegan, yoga-loving, meditating health junkie. But I had systemic inflammation, and autoimmune disorders are the result of your body fighting itself. It wasn't until I did an elimination cleanse and removed grains, legumes, dairy, and eggs that I realized they were all a problem for me. It even turns out that dairy and especially eggs are the worst culprits of them all. Today, I eat a lot of healthy fat and organic protein (including meat). My immune system is calm, and my blood work is normal. It has been a decade-long roller coaster to get to this point, with a lot of personal experimenting."

Um, whoa. Right? Doctors and fad diets did not help Megan correct her problems. Megan helped Megan. At best, keeping a food journal and then doing an elimination diet is a great way to clear your skin and help you find what is triggering your symptoms. If you are lucky enough not to have any, then it's a great way to clean up your whole system. You will absolutely notice results, and you will not be sorry.

CHAPTER 4

EAT LIKE YOUR SKIN DEPENDS ON IT

By this point you're already closer to having amazing skin than you were just a few weeks ago. You've kept a food journal and done an elimination diet, and when you see someone eating any of your newly discovered culprit foods, you feel an urge to slap it out of their hands. You feel as if you have all of the answers to life. That's awesome! Most of us are so in the dark about our diets and lifestyles that just stepping out into the light is a huge relief. You have information, you have better digestion, and you have better skin. So now you're in. You know how good you can feel, and you're more aware of the things that make you feel slightly off. (If you haven't kept your food journal and done your elimination yet, stop right here and go back to Chapter 3. I've got my eye on you. . . .)

Everything you've done up until this point has helped you establish a baseline for a healthy lifestyle. Now we're about to embark on a whole new phase in this journey, one in which you're going to raise your wellness to crazy new heights. Think of it this way: you know what causes your skin to act up, now you're not just going to avoid the breakouts/blotchiness/itchiness/redness/rashes, you're going to start finding what makes your skin radiant and glowing and angelic.

A FEW BASIC NUTRITION FACTS

You know that your diet is strongly tied to the state of your health (and therefore the state of your skin), so you've eliminated the bad stuff. Or at least, most of it, right? Now it's time to take a closer look at the good stuff. I like to wait until this stage to talk about vitamins and minerals and carbs and proteins and fats—aka, *micronutrients* and *macronutrients*—because, let's be honest: before you start worrying about your magnesium intake, I need you to stop eating donuts. But it's important to touch on it here, at least briefly, so you really understand how food affects your skin.

Macronutrients are carbohydrates, proteins, and fats. Macronutrients provide energy, and each has specific functions that keep you alive. Carbohydrates are our main source of energy and are needed for your brain, nervous system, kidney, and muscles. Proteins are necessary for growth, tissue repair, and a well-functioning immune system. Fats are the most energy-dense macronutrient, and they are responsible for normal growth and development, cellular health, and the absorption of fat-soluble vitamins. Big-picture discussions of nutrition focus on ratios of macronutrients in the diet: what percentage of our food intake should consist of carbs, fats, or proteins. Varying balances of these ratios are the premise for zillions of diet books.

Micronutrients are the vitamins and minerals contained in your macronutrients: minerals like copper, zinc, sodium, and magnesium, and vitamins like A, B, C, D, E, and K. You need very small amounts of micronutrients to survive, which is where the "micro" part comes in, but if you aren't getting enough of them, your body can't operate as efficiently as it should. And this book mostly exists because you're not getting enough of them.

Because they are packed with nutrients, healthy foods will contribute to clear, youthful skin while nutrient-depleted foods will do the opposite. We're going to keep this simple and talk only about the foods that make the biggest positive impact, and then we'll turn to some bad food habits that your food journal may have missed. Remember that even the things we discuss here must fit into the context of who you are. All nutrition science should be thought of as "mostly true"— meaning lots of studies support the general conclusions. But all science is in a constant state of evolution, and we learn new things about nutrition every day, some of which totally flies in the face of long-held truths. Remember, it wasn't that long ago that we thought it was perfectly fine to smoke while pregnant. Things change.

I don't love highlighting specific micronutrients for my clients because it kind of misses the point; vitamins and minerals must all work together to keep you alive. Without vitamin D, calcium cannot do its job. Without enough vitamin K_1, your body cannot get enough vitamin K_2. You cannot have a strong immune system by just getting more vitamin C; you can't fight free radicals by just taking some vitamin A; and you definitely can't get better skin by consuming only one specific vitamin or mineral. But all of that aside, everyone loves a handy chart. Plus, I think seeing it all mapped out shows you how surprisingly easy it is to get your correct dose each day. Include some healthy, whole foods, and you'll get the nutrients you need. Easy as that!

NUTRIENT[14]	BEST SOURCES	WHAT IT DOES IN YOUR BODY	WHAT IT DOES FOR YOUR SKIN
Vitamin A	Sweet potato, beef liver, spinach, carrots	Regulates cell growth	Reduces fine lines and wrinkles; prevents acne, UV damage, and dry skin
Vitamins B_6 and B_{12}	Tuna, chickpeas, beef liver, clams, salmon, sweet potato, potato, banana	Regulate how fat and protein are processed; help make DNA	Protect against cell damage and dehydration
Vitamin C	Raw red and green bell pepper, oranges, kiwis, broccoli	Essential to immune system function; protects against free radicals	Helps produce collagen; repairs tissue and sun damage
Vitamin D	Sunlight, salmon, sardines, egg yolks	Crucial for bone growth, nerve function, and immune health	Fights acne; aids in collagen production; reduces dark spots and wrinkles
Vitamin E	Almonds, sunflower seeds, peanuts, whole wheat, hazelnuts	Vital to immune function and vascular health	Prevents oxidative damage that leads to premature aging
Vitamins K_1 and K_2	Leafy greens and fermented foods; the normal processes of healthy gut bacteria	Needed for bone formation and vascular health	Promote elastin formation; helps heal bruises
Zinc	Oysters, beef, crab, yogurt, cashews	Essential to immune health and DNA and protein synthesis	Helps hair and nails grow; protects against infection and sun damage
Selenium	Brazil nuts, tuna, halibut, sardines, cottage cheese, brown rice	May help reduce the risk of some forms of cancer and cardiovascular disease	Helps repair UV radiation damage; protects against skin cancer
Calcium	Yogurt, sardines, milk, salmon, kale	Required for vascular, musculoskeletal, nervous system, and hormonal health	Helps with skin thickness and regulates skin cell production

Do you know which foods contain virtually no micro-nutrients? That's right—processed foods. Anything that comes in a box has a whole lot less nutrient value than something that comes from nature. I won't bother going into too much detail about why this category of "food" is bad for you and your skin, because there is plenty of evidence out there that chemically altered and synthesized food is not as good for you as natural food—and I think you are probably already aware of this. Just remember that synthetic foods are not recognized by your body as actual food (because they aren't). When your body struggles to process them, you become inflamed. Inflammation in the body leads to inflammation in the skin, which, as you know, is a beauty killer. Additionally, every time you miss an opportunity to eat nutrient-rich food, you are missing an opportunity to nourish and invigorate your skin.

Any time I hear about some "miraculous" new synthetic food additive, I think about Olestra. Do you remember Olestra? It was a fat-free fat substitute developed by Procter & Gamble and approved by the FDA for use in food in 1996, during the Great Fat-Free Diet Craze. It gave processed foods like potato chips that familiar greasy feel and crunch without adding any fat. It was the 1990s dieter's dream! The only problem was that it made it harder for your body to absorb actual nutrients, like vitamins A, D, E, and K, and it caused abdominal cramping . . . and anal leakage. Minor inconveniences. My point is, at their best, synthetic foods are devoid of nutrients and are doing nothing to help your skin. At their worst, they can have devastating side effects and health consequences. I don't even think of them as foods, and I'm not going to waste any more time on them here. You shouldn't, either.

One more thing: remember that you are now your own diet expert. You've done a lot of work to discover what does and doesn't work for you. If you uncovered a culprit in your food journal that was making you break out or giving you an itchy scalp and you see it listed in the coming pages as a recommended food that's great for your skin, *listen to your body*, not to me. Now that you have the knowledge of who you are, you also have your parameters. Take my recommendations and apply the parts that make sense for you.

THE GOOD FOODS LIST

Think of all good, nutrient-dense foods as superfoods—ingredients you want to incorporate into your diet frequently to keep your system running at its very best. Remember how I said your problem foods are kind of like a terrible ex? Well, these good foods are the opposite. They're the foods you want to commit to, the ones you should cuddle up with every night and marry.

Greens

Green leafy vegetables give you the most bang for your buck, literally and nutritionally, of any food out there. They're extremely affordable, and eating a wide variety of them every day gives you basically every micronutrient your body could ever need. Spinach alone contains at least thirteen different antioxidant and anticancer compounds. Greens in general have been proven to fight cancer, diabetes, arthritis, Alzheimer's, heart attack, stroke, high cholesterol, and heart disease. The high quantity of antioxidants in greens is especially important for your skin because antioxidants fight free radicals. But they also contain high levels of vitamin A, which fights acne and repairs damaged skin, as well as folate, beta-carotene, B vitamins, vitamin E, iron, calcium, magnesium, and potassium. All of the beauty vitamins and minerals. Greens are also high in anti-inflammatory flavonoids, which can act as antihistamines and antimicrobials in your body. They're like steroids for your immune system.

A Healthy Kitchen = A DIY Beauty Lab

The best part is how many greens are available to you. Don't waste your time worrying about which green is the best, just eat as many different kinds as you can. Kale is getting its fifteen minutes of fame right now—it seems to be in everything—but that does not mean arugula is not also awesome. Or chard. Or broccoli. If there's one you don't like, maybe it's steamed brussels sprouts (it's probably steamed brussels sprouts), skip it! There are plenty of other green vegetables to choose from and a million different ways to cook them. And the great thing is, they are all inexpensive, and getting enough of them in your diet to make a significant impact on your health is incredibly easy.

You may have read something on Facebook about a woman who got sick from eating too much raw kale. This is not something that should concern you or give you pause before ordering a kale salad. That lady was eating *a lot* of kale. (Didn't you learn while you were keeping your food journal that it's never a good idea to consume any one single food over and over every day?) You are most likely not eating like that lady. Trust me. If you have breakouts or splotchy skin, and between bites of hamburger you tell me, "I'm worried about my thyroid, are you sure I shouldn't eat less kale?" then I'm going to smack you.

Greens to aim for: Spinach, kale, collard, chard, red and green leaf lettuce, romaine lettuce, iceberg lettuce (yes, it's good for you), cabbage, bok choy, broccoli, mustard greens, turnip greens, beet greens, watercress, arugula, fennel, nettles, mint, and delicious brussels sprouts.

FAVORITE GREENS	ESPECIALLY HIGH IN . . .	TIPS AND BEST PRACTICES
Kale Lettuce (all types) Spinach Broccoli Brussels sprouts Cabbage Bok choy Mustard greens Turnip greens Beet greens Watercress Fennel Mint Nettles	Vitamins A, C, and K, and water, which promote the formation of elastin, heal bruises, help produce collagen, repair tissue and sun damage, reduce fine lines and wrinkles, and prevent acne, UV damage, and dry skin	De-stem and consume both raw and cooked greens regularly, add fat so that you feel full and to help you absorb fat-soluble vitamins. Always wash greens thoroughly to get rid of dirt and grit. Try to find organic greens that didn't have to travel too far to get to you; the fresher they are the more nutritious they are.

How to incorporate greens into your diet: Here are a few of my favorite greens, as well as simple ways to prepare them.

NETTLES: If you've ever touched fresh nettle, you know it can sting your skin. This sting, it turns out, seems to have a healing effect: nettles can be used topically to treat eczema and skin rashes. While your skin turns red and can start to hurt, the nettle is actually calming inflammation both topically (like your eczema) and internally (like your arthritis). If you're afraid of the sting, don't worry, cooking them takes it away. You can make nettle tea by bringing two parts water to one part nettles to a boil. Cool down and sip, or boil longer for a stronger brew. Apply the boiled leaves to your skin while you sip!

I also love to cook with nettles. Here's a recipe that takes minutes to prepare:

SIMPLE STINGING NETTLE SOUP

1 tablespoon grass-fed butter, olive oil, or coconut oil
1 onion, finely chopped
1 carrot, diced
1 stalk celery, finely chopped
1 to 2 large potatoes, cut into small chunks
Sea salt and pepper to taste
16 ounces low-sodium vegetable broth
1 to 3 cups of nettles, chopped
½ cup almond, dairy, coconut, or rice milk (optional)

Heat the butter, olive oil, or coconut oil in a large soup pot over medium heat until it is hot. Add the onion, carrot, celery, and potatoes. Add sea salt and pepper to taste. When onions are translucent and vegetables begin to soften, pour in the broth and bring to a boil. Turn the heat down to low and simmer, covered, until potatoes are soft, fifteen to twenty minutes. Add up to 3 cups of chopped fresh nettles and simmer for a few more minutes. Cool and blend with an immersion blender, crush veggies manually with the back of a spoon, or leave as is. (I think blended is the most yummy!) Stir in up to half a cup of your favorite milk to make it creamy.

KALE: There is actually good reason for kale getting so much glory these days. In addition to offering folate, magnesium, iron, quercetin (a powerful anti-inflammatory and anticancer compound), and other incredibly important vitamins and minerals, kale is also versatile to cook with and, when prepared properly, delicious. Kale needs a little bit of love to taste good. When it's not given this love, it's true deliciousness is hidden.

For my taste buds, the special key to good kale is removing the stems. The stems are tough to chew and have a completely different flavor from the leaf. Also, you don't have to feel guilty about not eating them because the leaves are where the most nutrients are hanging out. Kale stems suck. Toss them. An easy way to get rid of them is to hold the stem at its thickest part with one hand, and take the leaves in a loose fist with your other hand. Slide your fist hand quickly straight down, away from your gripping hand. The leaves will peel right away from the stem. Voilà!

Here are a few of my favorite ways to prepare kale:

1. Add 1 or 2 large leaves to a smoothie (you won't even notice it's there).
2. Kale chips are way, way cheaper to make than to buy, and insanely easy. Put washed and dried (and de-stemmed) leaves on a baking sheet and bake at 350° Fahrenheit for ten to fifteen minutes. That's it. You can flavor them however you want: olive oil, coconut oil, sea salt, nutritional yeast, parmesan cheese . . . Sprinkle these ingredients on the kale before it goes into the oven and again when it comes out.
3. Kale on the stove top takes longer to cook down and has a bit more flavor than spinach. It will end up slightly chewier, more like seaweed in texture than like lettuce. My favorite ways to flavor kale include different combinations of tamari, balsamic vinegar, coconut oil, garlic, and truffle oil.

Use these quick, simple recipes to prepare almost any green vegetable:

Sautéed Greens

1 tablespoon olive oil or grass-fed butter
1 head kale or chard, de-stemmed and shredded or hand-torn
1 tablespoon tamari soy sauce
1 tablespoon balsamic vinegar

Heat about a tablespoon of olive oil or grass-fed butter in a pan over medium heat. Add a head of shredded or hand-torn, de-stemmed kale or chard (or chopped bok choy or any other green vegetable you like) and stir until bright green and wilted. Place it in a bowl and drizzle with a tablespoon of tamari soy sauce and a tablespoon of balsamic vinegar (or a little more, depending on your taste). Mix well. Dig in.

Roasted Greens

1 head broccoli, chopped, or ½ pound brussels sprouts,
    chopped
2 tablespoons oil, grass-fed butter, or ghee
Sea salt and pepper to taste

Preheat your oven to 350°F. Place a head of chopped broccoli or brussels sprouts onto a cookie sheet. Drizzle with olive oil or melted butter or ghee (clarified butter), add a teaspoon of sea salt and a pinch of black pepper, and mix until everything is well coated. Roast for fifteen to twenty minutes, stirring several times during roasting. If you're making brussels sprouts, roast until they're soft when you pierce them with a fork. The time will vary, depending on your oven, but the veggies will become brighter and slightly crispy on the outside. To kick up the flavor, add a squeeze of lemon or a (tiny) sprinkle of cheese over your veggies!

Fatten Up Your Veggies

You may have noticed that I like to add oil or butter to my greens. I do this for a few reasons, the most obvious being that it makes them taste better. Much better. This is tied to the second reason, which is that adding fat to your veggies makes them significantly more satiating. You'll actually get full from eating vegetables, which is kind of like a mini-miracle the first time you experience it. Take it from my nutritionist friend Andy Bellatti, MS, RD: "It's always important to eat some healthful fats (think avocados, nuts, seeds, olive/coconut oil) with vegetables since some nutrients, including vitamins A, D, E, and K, and healthful antioxidants—such as carotenoids—can only be absorbed by our bodies with the help of fat. Put away that fat-free salad dressing!" So fat is especially important with greens, since they are highest in vitamins A and K. Plus, fat-free salad dressing is not nearly as delicious as full-fat dressing.

Fruit

With all of the (well-deserved) bad press that sugar is getting these days, it's a sad time for fruit. There really aren't any fruit publicists out there fighting the good fight for grapes and oranges and pineapples. Lots of us are starting to think that fruit is as damaging for our waistlines and skin as Twinkies and soda. But fruit is second only to greens as the most nutrient-packed beauty superfood. It's true that fruit contains a lot of sugar (in the form of fructose), but the key difference between the sugar in fruit and the sugar you stir into your coffee is something called fiber. (For the record, the sugar in Twinkies and soda is only a distant cousin of the sugar in fruit—it's high-octane, man-made sugar on steroids.)

Fiber is what helps your body process all of the food you eat and expel all of the waste you don't need. Fiber lessens the negative impact of sugar on your body, and the large amount of fiber in fruit helps your body in a variety of ways. It fills you up, keeps your energy level stable, and aids digestion. Even *fresh* juice contains enough fiber to be really great for your system. Fresh juice is very different from the "dead" fruit juice in your grocery store aisle—that stuff has been heated to kill all the bacteria (and with it, the nutrients), filtered to remove all of the fiber, and beefed up with fake sugars and colors and flavors to mimic the original. That is not the kind of fruit I'm encouraging you to eat. But you know this. Remember what I said earlier about real food versus fake food? Okay, great.

Fruit is also extremely hydrating and filling, and a nice fruit snack is a super-effective way of dealing with sugar cravings. It can be hard at first to swap out your sugary favorites for a nice apple or a few chunks of melon, especially when you're used to the Franken-sweets that your brain and body are slightly addicted to, but once you start eating fruit regularly, you'll find that you crave it.

Fruit to aim for: whole, fresh fruit or fruit juices made in a blender or juicer. Not the fruit juice from the grocery store.

FAVORITE FRUITS	ESPECIALLY HIGH IN...	TIPS AND BEST PRACTICES
Apples Pears Papayas Mangos Berries Bananas Grapes Cherries Lemons Oranges Grapefruits Avocados Tomatoes	Vitamin C and fiber, which help produce collagen, repair tissue, and heal sun damage	Fruit can upset some people's digestion if eaten with other foods, so have it alone if you think you may fall in this category. Generally the part of the fruit closest to the peel is the healthiest, so eat the white parts on your citrus and scoop your avocado. Opt for organic, especially for fruits that have a thin peel or no peel.

How to incorporate fruit into your diet: Try having a fruit salad first thing in the morning. Because fruit is high in fiber, eating it in the morning actually helps to keep your blood sugar stable throughout the day; therefore, you'll be less likely to binge on snacks and sweets later. Plus, it's incredibly common for people to skip breakfast, and fruit is a light and easy way to get your body going. Eating fruit for breakfast will help kick-start your digestion and metabolism in the morning—like an alarm clock for your insides. Pick whatever fruit you like the most and eat enough to get full. Remember good-for-you fiber helps you process the fructose. And a bowl of the sweetest fruit is still a superfood, while that coffee crumb cake can't compete.

IF YOU HAD TO add just one fruit to your diet, pick papaya. Papaya is a superfruit for your skin. It fights aging, heals sunburn, removes dead skin cells, soothes irritation, fights breakouts, and brightens the skin. And it's especially helpful after a rough food moment—like when you went on vacation and ate all of your food culprits in one meal, then again in another, then another. Try having a few bites of papaya right after you eat the bad foods. The enzymes will help your belly break them down much faster and more easily, and they'll remain in your body for a shorter time, which means they'll do less damage. Papaya is great with a squeeze of lime. Or you can mash up a little and apply it to your face as a mask. Leave it on for up to twenty minutes and rinse off for brighter, softer skin.

IF YOU ABSOLUTELY HATE eating fruit, juice or blend it. Or buy a fresh juice or a fresh fruit smoothie. It's possible there is nothing better in the world than fresh fruit juice. And in a blender with some ice, strawberries, bananas, mango, blueberries . . . I mean, I can't even think of a sweet fruit that isn't delicious when blended or juiced. If you're new to the juicing/smoothie experience, let the experts at your local juice bar help you select a good combination. I've worked in juice bars and can attest that my coworkers really knew how to create delicious drinks. You don't have to choose some exotic blend of goji berries and maca powder and all sorts of things you've never heard of. Start with the fruit that sounds awesome to you and branch out into adding veggies when you're ready. Carrots and beets are two sweet vegetables that are easy to add to fruit juice and will boost the nutrient level through the roof.

A Great Shake

Sarma Melngailis is royalty in the raw-food world. She created the acclaimed plant-based restaurant Pure Food and Wine in New York City and also owns One Lucky Duck, which sells amazing foods in store and online. It just so happens she also used to be my boss. This is a woman who knows how to make a seriously delicious and nutritious smoothie, so I asked her to share her secrets. (Sarma hates the word *smoothie*, though, so she calls her creations *shakes*.) Here are her tips for creating skin-boosting shakes that will give you angelic skin while also tasting divine:

The basics: cucumber, citrus, coconut water. To that you'll add in fruit and greens. Cucumber is hydrating, and coconut water is full of electrolytes. These are two of the most perfect hydrating foods. Berries are full of antioxidants, and greens are full of vitamins and protein. You don't need to measure out exact amounts, just adjust as you go. Too thick? Add more water. Not sweet enough? Add more fruit.

One simple recipe: in a blender, add approximately one peeled and chopped cucumber. Cut the peel away from a grapefruit, lemon, lime, or all three. Roughly chop and add maybe half the grapefruit, half the lemon, and half the lime. Then pour in some coconut water. You can also use filtered tap water. Then blend this into a smooth liquid. (A Vitamix or high-speed blender will make these shakes really smooth, but if you have only a regular old blender, that's fine, too, just blend a little longer. The shake will be a little less smooth.) This is your shake base.

To this base, add fruits and greens. My favorite fruits to add are pineapple and mango, ideally both. They have tart flavors and pair well with greens. You can also add herbs—cilantro, parsley, or mint. Or you don't have to use any herbs at all. Just add a few leaves of kale (stems removed), Swiss chard, a handful of spinach leaves, or any lettuces you like. Keep in mind, some greens are mild, some more bitter. So taste as you go, and you'll get to know how much you're comfortable with.

If you're not ready for greens or don't have any on hand, add fresh berries to the shake base. Blackberries, blueberries . . . they're among the highest antioxidant foods (i.e., good for your health and skin).

With the basics, you can really do whatever you want. Have fresh peaches? Add those! Honeydew melon? Toss that in. A little banana is great, too (it adds a little creaminess, and, if frozen, a nice chill). All you need to keep in mind is balancing the sweet, the green, and the citrus. And, if appearance matters to you, consider the color of what you add. Strawberries or any red fruit in a shake along with greens will make the color a bit muddy-looking. It'll taste delicious, but if you're making it for a friend, you may want to keep it pretty. That's why I love mango and pineapple with greens, it keeps everything bright.

One of the best add-ins for clear skin is aloe vera juice. I often add a splash to my shakes.

Fat

Fat is even more controversial than fruit. Leave it to me to give you only scandalous food recommendations. Hopefully by now, you've heard some of the new evidence proving that our time spent obsessively cutting fat from our diets has not benefited us in any way. In fact, it's done the opposite. I believe that all the years we spent cutting fat from (and adding carbs and sugars to) our diet have contributed to our epidemic levels of health problems today—as well as the rise in nagging skin ailments like eczema and psoriasis. Eating fat is absolutely essential to maintaining good health, and it is crucial to having amazing skin.

Honestly, I think the word *fat* itself is part of the problem, because people tend to confuse dietary fat with body fat. The fat inside your body is a completely different thing than the fat you consume in your diet. Fat cells do not necessarily come from or grow in size as a result of eating fat. Fat cells grow in response to a very complicated process, regulated by hormones, and influenced by everything you eat (but especially sugar). In fact, with very rare exceptions, fat cells are produced in your body only twice in your life: while you're a fetus, and while you're in puberty. The rest of your life, they are only shrinking or growing in size. Most of a man's fat is in his chest and belly. Most of a woman's fat is in her breasts, hips, waist, and butt. The difference is due to estrogen and testosterone levels, which are responsible for producing the fat cells for your body during puberty.

The fat that you *eat* helps your body regulate energy by providing a backup if your sugar supply runs out. Fat is also responsible for processing fat-soluble vitamins, which include A, D, E, and K (see page 72 for more information). These vitamins are stored in your liver and fatty tissues, and, without dietary fat, your body wouldn't be able to use them. You may remember from our macronutrient discussion that fats are actually more energy-dense than protein and carbs, which means the energy fat gives you will last longer than that from protein and carbs.

The body can create some of the fats it needs to survive, but there are other fats essential to life that you can get only from food sources. These are called essential fatty acids (EFAs), also known as omega-3 and omega-6 fatty acids. These fats are critical to helping your body produce healthy cells, including skin cells. They also aid in the production of sebum, which, as you know, keeps your skin hydrated and looking youthful. If you're not getting enough fat, you will experience both dryness and inflammation. You will also be more sensitive to sunlight, more prone to breakouts, and more likely to develop psoriasis. Lack of adequate fat in the diet is also linked to symptoms like arthritis, low energy, and mood swings. And eating the wrong proportion of omegas or lots of low-quality dietary fat (like factory-farmed dairy and fried oils) which will lead to an overproduction of sebum, which will cause you to breakout.

The only way to get EFAs is through your diet, which means that you are in complete control of how much of this critical building block your body is getting. But it's important to note that EFAs have to be consumed in the right ratio for your body to get what it needs. Processed foods are full of omega-6s, and when you consume too many omega-6s and not enough omega-3s, inflammation runs rampant in the body. And you remember our chat about inflammation, right? Not only is it linked to many deadly diseases, in skin terms, it is the underlying condition for acne, psoriasis, rosacea, and many others.

So how do you get the right ratio of these magical omegas? Easy. Natural, whole, fatty foods have them in the right proportion already. Naturally. Did I mention they're natural?

Fats to aim for: coconut products (oil, milk, cream, butter), olive oil, organic butter and ghee, avocado, flax, nuts, and seeds.

FAVORITE FATS	ESPECIALLY HIGH IN ...	TIPS AND BEST PRACTICES
Coconuts Olive oil Organic butter and ghee Organic eggs Avocados Flax Almonds Brazil nuts	Omegas and vitamin E, which prevent oxidative damage that leads to premature aging	Coconut products are a great way to cut back on dairy. Fats have omegas in different proportions, as well as small amounts of additional micronutrients, so eat a variety. Cook with thicker oils like coconut oil and butter; put thinner oils like olive oil on raw foods or already-cooked food.

How to incorporate fats into your diet: Here is my list of favorite sources of fat, along with some of my favorite ways to eat them!

COCONUT OIL: This delicious oil is special among plant fats because it has a high concentration of what are called medium-chain-length fatty acids, which are much easier for your body to digest than other types of fats. Coconut oil helps your body fight viruses and bacteria, improves your metabolism, and reduces inflammation. It's also great to cook with, since it can withstand a lot of heat without breaking down and creating free radicals like some other oils do. And it's delicious on popcorn! In the good old days, movie popcorn and Ritz crackers were both made with coconut oil. Somewhere along the line, however, they decided to switch to partially hydrogenated fats (aka, trans fats). Hopefully, we'll get it right again soon! Here's a quick and super-delicious way to get some healthy fat and fiber in one delicious snack.

Coco-Popcorn

3 tablespoons extra-virgin coconut oil
½ cup organic popcorn kernels
Sea salt to taste
Hot sauce, paprika, nutritional yeast, or your favorite topping

Add coconut oil to a large, deep pot and place over medium high heat. When oil is hot, add corn kernels and cover, continuing to cook on medium-high, making sure to shake the pot on the burner as the kernels begin to pop to help them pop evenly. Hold the lid slightly ajar to avoid a messy kitchen and to allow some steam to escape. Pull the pot off the burner as soon as the popping slows. Once it's off the burner, cover it for another thirty seconds while any remaining kernels pop. Sprinkle with sea salt and add your favorite toppings. I know, it's really good.

OLIVE OIL: This popular oil contains the highest level of mono-unsaturated fat (aka, unsaturated fat) of any plant oil. It lowers cholesterol, fights inflammation, lowers blood pressure, promotes weight loss, and reduces your risk for developing diabetes, arthritis, and osteoporosis. And it's extremely high in vitamin E, which fights premature aging. Olive oil is best when unrefined, so always look for extra-virgin and drizzle on raw veggies or on food after it's been cooked to preserve the nutritional integrity of the oil.

HOMEMADE MAYO

1 egg yolk (organic)
1 teaspoon white wine vinegar
½ teaspoon Dijon mustard
½ teaspoon sea salt (or more to taste)
¾ cup olive oil
Juice of half a lemon

You'll need an immersion blender for this recipe. Place all ingredients in a tall glass or jar that is just wide enough for your stick blender to reach the bottom completely. Give it one quick pulse, then another. You'll see the ingredients start to blend together and turn white. Give it a few more pulses until it's mostly white, then turn the blender on completely and move it in an up-and-down motion. Done. Fresh, raw, wholesome mayonnaise. Store in the fridge for up to one week.

GRASS-FED ORGANIC BUTTER: High-quality, organic, grass-fed butter is one of the best sources of vitamin K_2, which helps your body to absorb and use calcium from food. Recent studies have called into question the old claim that saturated fats lead to an increased risk of heart disease, so you no longer need to be scared of butter.[15] Like coconut oil, it contains medium-chain triglycerides, which are easy for the body to break down and use. Butter is also high in vitamins A, D, and E, as well as many minerals, which means that it promotes wound healing and protects against blood clots. It's also high in conjugated linoleic acid, or CLA, which has been shown to help reduce body fat. So basically, grass-fed butter makes you skinny. (Remember, I'm not talking about gross industrial butter. That will for sure not make you skinny or healthy or anything good.)

I really racked my brain to think of a way to use grass-fed butter that would be new to you, and here's what I came up with: Buttered coffee. If you haven't heard about this new underground health craze, here's what you do: add 1 teaspoon of grass-fed butter (and 1 teaspoon of coconut oil, if you're really feeling it) to a hot cup of coffee in the morning. Put it in a blender or just mix it the best you can. I like to add a touch of raw honey also. You might think it sounds crazy (I did at first, too), but it's actually really delicious, and the mix of healthy fats first thing in the morning helps stabilize your appetite and energize you throughout your day.

Why Organic?

Just like many nutrients are stored in fatty tissue, so are pesticides, insecticides, and other chemicals. That is not true just for humans; it is also true for animals. That means when you eat meat or dairy, you are consuming everything that has been stored in an animal's body. Organic meat is free of many, many chemicals used in conventional cattle raising. Additionally, these days animals raised in a factory farm are not fed food that is easy for them to digest, and most are living in horrible conditions, so they are also fed antibiotics to keep them healthy. All of that is a part of what's on your plate; it doesn't just go away once it's wrapped in cellophane. I call this "sad meat." Eat happy meat and dairy instead. Look for the USDA organic logo or, better yet, the grass-fed, free-range goodies at your local farmers market.

AVOCADO: Believe it or not, avocado is a fruit! A beautiful and delicious one with a really high content of fat. Avocados contain phytonutrients called carotenoids, which are incredibly powerful anti-inflammatories. They also help make the nutrients in raw vegetables more available to your body to use, so they're a great thing to throw in a salad. They are also super-high in vitamin E and fiber. The most nutritious part of an avocado is right under the peel, so be sure to use a spoon to scoop out the "meat" closest to the peel!

My favorite way to eat avocado is by whipping up some avocado toast. It makes a great breakfast or afternoon snack. Just mash up a half an avocado and spread it over a piece of toast. Sprinkle with salt, pepper, and a splash of lemon or hot sauce. Mmm!

SARDINES: Okay, so sardines are intense, on multiple levels. You probably don't eat many of them because of their strong flavor, but I urge you to give them a chance, because they are so good for you. Sardines are extremely high in omega-3s (a can of sardines offers you a lot more omega-3 power than a fish oil pill), vitamin B_{12}, vitamin D, and selenium, which are basically all of the nutrients you need for beautiful skin, all in one place! They are an oily fish, and you may have heard of the importance of fish oils in your diet, or as a supplement. Bigger fish can contain a higher concentration of pollutants because they are higher on the food chain, so smaller fish, like sardines (and mackerel and anchovies) are a better choice. Eating smaller fish also means that you can enjoy them more often than is recommended for other types of fish. My favorite way to eat them is blended into a creamy homemade dressing.

HOMEMADE CAESAR DRESSING

1 cup olive oil mayo
1–2 canned sardines or anchovies
2 cloves garlic, peeled
Juice of half a lemon
1 tablespoon white wine vinegar
Sea salt and plenty of black pepper to taste

Place all ingredients in a blender and blend until creamy. Use as a dressing for your favorite greens (it's really delicious on chopped romaine), or use as a dip for roasted veggies like brussels sprouts.

Fermented Foods

Do you eat cheese? Sourdough bread? Yogurt? Drink beer or wine? Okay, great, then you are already familiar with fermented foods. My clients are always terrified of fermented foods, and it takes a lot of convincing before they understand that so much of what they're eating already is fermented.

Before our society got pasteurization-happy, even more food was just swimming in bacteria. And that food was better for us then than it is now.

Pasteurization may keep us safer in some ways (it kills bad bacteria and prevents spoilage), but our fear of outside bacteria is a little misguided. While some bacteria is dangerous, much of it is actually beneficial to our immune systems. In fact, new research shows that kids who live in naturally dirty environments (think farms with animals or outdoor pets that like to cuddle) end up with stronger immune systems as adults.[16] Healthy, thriving bacterial ecosystems that live on our skin and in our intestines are part of what keep us healthy. People missing these crucial bacteria in their gut have digestive problems and allergies.

There are actually trillions of microorganisms in your gut, making up what is known as your microbiome. The research on the human microbiome is still very new but also very powerful. Your gut flora support the healthy functioning of everything from your digestive tract to your immune system and from your heart to your brain. Babies with a high amount of gut flora are less likely to develop eczema or asthma later in life. Some studies have shown that when these essential microbes are introduced into the gut, people get healthier and lose weight without making any other lifestyle changes.

And importantly for you, people with healthy bacteria on their skin break out less often than people with less bacteria. Studies have shown that people with clear skin have 20 percent more bacteria production than those with acne. Researchers are working on a topical bacterial product that you can apply to your skin to actually *clean* it. I mean, it's amazing really. And it's a huge missing link in our health and our skin's health. We make it tough on our bodies to keep healthy levels of bacteria on the inside and outside with our excessive use of antibiotics, which kill all the bacteria in our guts in one fell swoop, and then with our obsession with pasteurization, which kills the bacteria in our food. But we can nourish our guts by adding probiotics (live, healthy microorganisms) and fermented foods.

But Jamie Lee Curtis Says . . .

Yes, there are healthy bacteria in yogurt, which is why you see so many commercials about women who love yogurt for their "regularity." But yogurt is not the best source of bacteria for a few reasons. The first is that it's dairy, whether or not it's fermented. And dairy—especially conventional, factory-farmed dairy—is a problem food for a lot of people. Second, yogurt is often full of added sugar, which defeats the healthy benefit. Lastly, because it's a processed food, you'd better believe it's not made the way your grandmama would have made it. If your grocery store has organic, grass-fed natural yogurt that you can eat plain (or better yet, if you can, make your own), then go for it! But I think of that sugary yogurt that comes in cups as nothing but a weird, synthetic probiotic supplement.

Fermented foods to aim for: Sauerkraut, tempeh, kimchee, miso, kombucha, kefir, and unsweetened natural yogurts.

FAVORITE FERMENTED FOODS	ESPECIALLY HIGH IN...	TIPS AND BEST PRACTICES
Sauerkraut Tempeh Kimchee Miso Kombucha Kefir Unsweetened yogurts	Probiotics, which reduce acne, fight inflammation, and help your skin heal more quickly	Overcooking a fermented food will kill its helpful bacteria. You can't get too much of this good thing, so *if* you add a little bit of each of these foods to your diet, you'll notice a big difference. And yes, it's true, probiotic foods will also help your regularity.

How to incorporate fermented foods into your diet: Unpasteurized sauerkraut and salt-brined pickles are amazing fermented foods that offer probiotic benefits. If you buy them prepared, make sure they're sitting in a refrigerated section, not on the shelf. Look for a label that says something like: "cabbage, salt" or "cabbage, carrots, salt, spices" or "cucumbers, salt" and nothing else. No vinegar, additives, or preservatives. Better yet, ferment your own sauerkraut on your kitchen counter. I swear it's easy and super-healthy and actually delicious.

COUNTER 'KRAUT

1 head cabbage
1 to 2 tablespoons sea salt

1. Cut a cabbage into quarters and cut out the core. Peel off the outer cabbage leaves and any leaves with black spots, and save one or two whole, unblemished leaves. Finely shred the remaining cabbage.

MAKING your own COUNTER KRAUT

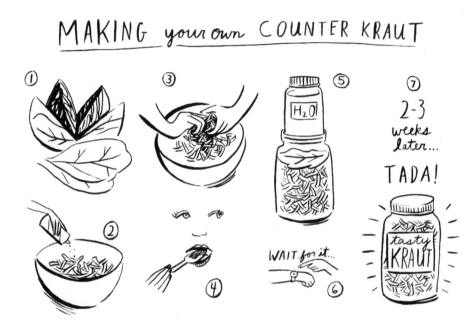

2. Put the shredded cabbage into a large bowl or pot and add 1 to 2 tablespoons of sea salt, depending on the size of your cabbage. An average one will need about 2 tablespoons, but if it's your first time, start with 1 tablespoon (you can add more later). One note: don't use iodized salt. Iodine will kill your fermentation.

3. After you add the salt, start breaking up the cabbage by "massaging" it, meaning: grab fistfuls of it and squeeze it, punch it, and just basically manhandle it. What you're doing is causing the cell walls to break apart while the salt pulls water from inside the cabbage. If your wrists and forearms start to ache, you're doing it right. In a couple of minutes, it will start to produce liquid. After five or ten minutes, your cabbage will look wilted and reduced in size, and there should be quite a lot of water in the bottom of your bowl (this is your "brine").

4. Once your cabbage is all mushy, get a clean fork to taste it for saltiness. (Make sure to avoid putting a dirty fork in your cabbage—you want to keep as much foreign bacteria out as you can.) If it tastes just a little too salty for your normal taste, then it's perfect. You want the 'kraut to be saltier than a normal meal should be, but not so salty that it's inedible.

5. Once it's ready, put it in a bowl or jar that's small enough that you can pack it tightly with your fist and deep enough that the liquid can rise up an inch or so above the surface of the shredded cabbage. A wide-mouth Mason jar is perfect for this. Now, you'll use the whole, unblemished cabbage leaves that you saved earlier to lay across the top of the chopped cabbage to hold down stray pieces under the liquid. You'll need a weight to keep the cabbage underwater. I fill a smaller jar with water and tightly cap it (so the water doesn't spill into your brine). Make sure to wash the outside of this second jar because it'll be touching the cabbage. The whole point here is to keep the cabbage submerged under the brine. This is an anaerobic fermentation, meaning it happens only when it's not exposed to oxygen, but gas needs to be able to escape so don't cover the whole jar with anything thicker than a cheesecloth.

6. Now set your counter 'kraut aside for a few days. How long is really a question of taste. It'll be slightly fermented in as few as three days. But if you want to be really hard-core, you can leave it for two or three weeks. Although—take it from me—it'll start stinking up your kitchen by that point. One thing to note: it is possible to get some mold on the surface of your brine if you're leaving it for a couple weeks. Just skim it off the top. Not a big deal at all. Like I said, sauerkraut is pretty much foolproof.

7. Now the best part! When you're ready, just take out the weighing jar and the cabbage leaves (skim off any mold and

seriously don't worry about it, it's totally safe), and put a lid on your 'kraut. It'll store in the fridge for a really long time (up to several months) if you make sure to scoop it out only with clean utensils. Not that you'll need to store it very long. Trust me, you'll be putting this stuff on everything. I add it to salads, veggie burgers, sausages, and as a topping on veggie soups. It's even amazing by itself as a simple side.

Spices

A friend of mine is a vegan chef who gets really upset when she hears people say that vegan food can't taste good. She always says, "Vegan food is great if you cook dirty." By which she means using a *lot* of flavorful herbs and spices. She cooks very dirty, and her food is incredible.

I love, love, love this idea of "cooking dirty." It's the perfect way to describe all of the amazingly fragrant foods that get largely ignored in the American diet—foods like garlic, ginger, turmeric, oregano, basil, curry, fennel, cardamom, cloves, and cinnamon. Black pepper and hot peppers. Sea salt. Herbs and spices are not only delicious, they are nutrient powerhouses.

All of these flavor boosters have tremendous health and skin benefits. They increase blood flow and circulation; they are packed with vitamins and minerals; they fight inflammation; they improve your body's ability to fight free radicals; they help create a stronger UV shield in your skin; they promote the production of collagen; and they make your skin less sensitive from the inside out. In the same way that they excite your taste buds, they stimulate your cells to function better. So eat dirty. It's so easy and it makes eating way, way more interesting.

FAVORITE "SPICES"	ESPECIALLY HIGH IN . . .	TIPS AND BEST PRACTICES
Garlic Ginger Turmeric Oregano Basil Curry Fennel Cardamom Cinnamon Thyme Cloves Bay leaves	Vitamin C, copper, iron, magnesium, and zinc, which increase blood flow and circulation, fight inflammation, fight free radicals, protect skin against UV damage, promote production of collagen, and make the skin less sensitive	Fresh is best, so try to use fresh garlic, ginger, turmeric, basil, and oregano if you can find them. Some spices can take getting used to for your digestive system, so if you're new to cooking dirty, start light. Taste as you go! It's the best way to know when you like how much you've added.

One of my favorite ways to dirty up my food is with my Put-It-On-Everything Spice Mix: combine 1 teaspoon each of cumin, paprika, oregano, basil, onion powder, garlic powder, black pepper, and turmeric with ½ teaspoon of salt and as much cayenne or chili powder as you want. Mix well. Put on everything: beef, fish, chicken, eggs, tofu, tempeh, greens, and beans.

Water

Flip open basically any lady magazine ever printed and you'll find a feature on your health or beauty with the same advice: drink water. I've decided magazines do this on purpose because—since most people think they drink plenty of water—it makes readers feel good before they get to the stuff they're for sure not doing. They see that first tip and they're like, "I'm so on top of this! I don't even have to finish reading this article. I bet I have clear skin and I just don't know it. Let me go check to make sure." Then they go look in the mirror and get bummed out.

102 • Skin Cleanse

This is one of the few times I will tell you to stop ignoring the lady-magazine advice! You think you're the world's best water drinker, but you're not. You are absolutely underhydrated, I can tell from here. Here's how you can tell: chapped lips, urine that's not completely or almost completely clear, trouble going poo, frequent headaches, being hungry all the time, anxiety symptoms, feeling dizzy, and having crazy dips in energy. Oh, and dry skin that stays dry no matter how much you drench it in moisturizer.

There has been some debate in the wellness community about the exact amount of water we should all be drinking. Ignore all the details. It's too much information, and all it does is confuse you so you end up doing nothing. Unless you are an Ironwoman or looking to become the next Williams sister, you do not need to micromanage your water intake. Just drink more, period. Cancer patients are often told to drink a gallon of water a day to flush the chemotherapy toxins from their systems. A gallon! That's an extreme example, but it makes you think about how many toxins we could all get rid of by just upping the amount of water we drink.

Drinking more water is also a way to make healthy eating easier. It is like pushing the Reset button for your body. If you increase how much of it you drink, you will feel better, your cravings will subside, and your skin will look better. And this is all without doing anything else! Here are some super-simple tips about your water intake that you *should* be thinking about:

- Diet Coke does not count. Do you understand this? Please read this tip over and over and over until you do. In fact, dark and caffeinated beverages in general do not count. They make you need more water. Sorry, but it's true. For every cup of coffee or soda you drink, you should add two cups of water to your day.

- Herbal teas and veggie juices do count.
- You can't live on herbal tea and veggie juice alone, so carry water around with you. Always have it handy, even if you never touch it (you will).
- Double fist your wineglass (or any other drink for that matter) with a glass of water.
- The receptacle matters. Personally, I have a bad attitude about water—I hate drinking it. But then I bought this adult sippy cup—a big cup with a built-in straw—and something about it makes me guzzle water. Find your sippy cup, and get attached to it.
- Don't stress too much about temperature, either. I know your yoga teacher said to drink warm water with lemon first thing in the morning. Do that if you like it. If you like iced water, drink that. If you like water with cucumber or oranges, frozen and then chopped up, consumed only while upside down, drink that. It doesn't really matter how you drink it, *just drink it.*

Supplements

The sad thing about supplements is that so many of them have very little evidence to show that they work. The even sadder thing about them is that most of us just ignore the idea of supplements altogether. Generally my clients fall into one of two categories: they either take the same multivitamin their mom's been giving them for years; or they take fifteen different things but, like, you know, when they remember. They have no idea why they're taking them, and they feel no real difference when they do or don't take them. Then there are a few outliers: people who very diligently and carefully supplement . . . but they don't feel much of a difference, either.

First of all, a supplement alone will not give you clear skin. It will also not give you younger skin. In fact, no supplement can ever solve any skin (or other) problem completely. It's just not the right way to think about supplements in general. They are meant to *supplement* what you are already doing. Like eating right, drinking lots of water, exercising, and taking care of your skin. Do all that, and you will help the supplements help you, which is all they're supposed to do. They're not magical.

And as my naturopath friend Laurie Brodsky, ND, puts it, "Just as important as it is with your food, reading the ingredient list on your supplements will help you make a wiser decision with regards to what you put into your body. You are what you eat (and absorb in your gut!), so be sure to choose a product devoid of artificial ingredients and from a company that shares with you full disclosure of their sourcing and ingredients."

But obviously my favorite supplements are just a little bit magical. Otherwise, I wouldn't recommend them. You're not ever going to hear me recommend a vitamin A pill or a skin supplement or—oh my God—garlic *pills?!* Apple cider vinegar *pills?* Avocado *pills?* Eat your vitamins, please.

Here are a few supplements I really like:

1. Probiotics. Because the truth is that you probably are not going to eat enough tempeh or 'kraut or miso to get the

amount of good bacteria that you need, and processed foods are killing it off anyway. Take a probiotic on an empty stomach and everything will work better, and you won't have to try as hard to drink fermented tea that smells like dirty socks.

2. Digestive enzymes. More than likely, you won't ever find out what's causing every stomachache you get, or every breakout, or every bout of itchy skin, but also more than likely, it is because foods that you can't pinpoint aren't being processed by your body correctly. Digestive enzymes help your belly do that work when it's struggling on its own. My favorites are full-spectrum enzyme capsules and papaya chewables. Both options work really quickly on an upset stomach, and they can help ease the discomfort a meal may cause if you take them before eating.

3. Greens powder. You need greens and/or vegetables at every single meal. And not, like, as a side dish, but as the largest part of the meal. Probably you are not doing that. An organic greens powder gives you a little boost, like a greens juice or a smoothie. Greens powder is fast and easy, and often packed with extra nutrients from foods you'd rarely eat otherwise, like açai berries and maca powder. Trust me, they're all good for you and for your skin.

4. Vitamin D. Listen to Dr. Laurie Brodsky: "Vitamin D, with all of its hormone-like, healing, and protective properties, is in my opinion, one of the most important supplements that we should all consider taking daily, especially through long winter seasons. I personally prefer liquid drops or an emulsified form of Vitamin D

for enhanced absorption, and always take it with a meal with some fat, since it is a fat-soluble vitamin."

Vitamin D is the only supplement where I break my rule because I think it is so, so, so important. Obviously, none of us would need to supplement it if we were getting enough sun, but it's nearly impossible to know whether you've crossed the fine line between healthy exposure and unhealthy, so as a society we've gotten afraid of the sun. Whether or not we're right to be, avoiding the sun completely is making us suffer internally. Recent studies point toward the conclusion that we are all at least a little vitamin D deficient. Get tested if you want proof, but for your skin, it's better to make sure you're getting enough.

GOING THROUGH A ROUGH food patch where you keep eating foods that mess up your stomach and skin? Take these supplements. Traveling so much that it's hard for you to stick to your routine? Take these supplements. Feeling "off"? Take these supplements. Starting to think you could just skip all of my other dietary advice and take these pills and some multivitamins and still look awesome and feel great? Trust me, it ain't gonna happen.

THE BAD FOODS LIST

Now that you've successfully added all of these good foods into your diet, it's important to stay vigilant to some of the little slipups that can creep back in to undermine your progress. There are a few bad habits that plague almost everyone I've ever worked with and can sometimes fall through the cracks when you're looking at your food journal. I want to point them out so that you can identify them and nip them in the bud before they become an issue!

That Milk/Cream/Half-and-Half in Your Morning Coffee

Here's the thing about dairy. I know that it's really common in the wellness community for dairy to be singled out as an evil food group. People claim that it makes your body too acidic, and it's the root cause of lots of our diseases, and we're all secretly allergic to it, and it disrupts your hormones, etc. I disagree with all of that. In fact, there is virtually no scientific evidence that dairy, in and of itself, is inherently evil.

But, wait! Most dairy *these days* is not the dairy of yester-year. It's not even really dairy anymore. It's a synthetic copy, like a junk-food version of the real thing. First of all, milk is homogenized, which stops it from ever separating, and then pasteurized, which, as we've discussed, kills virtually all of the bacteria it contains. And then there's the way most dairy cows are raised: they're fed hormones and antibiotics, which end up in their milk and then in your body. (Think about your last friend who breast-fed and how crazy she was about everything she put in her body. Hormones? Drugs? Not in her milk.)

Hormones affect your skin. Antibiotics kill the good bacteria in your body, which affects your skin. Industrialized dairy, in general, does many things to give us bad skin. The one and only thing that every individual I've ever known with perfectly clear skin has in common is that they eat no dairy. And maybe you don't want to hear this, but they are fanatical about it. No butter, no cheese, no milk, no cream, no yogurt.

They are either lactose intolerant or they behave as if they are. Dairy is just not an option for them.

So if you are suffering from breakouts as an adult, you may want to reconsider that daily latte habit.

That Soy Milk in Your Morning Coffee

I know! I just told you to stop adding milk to your coffee, and now I go and take away your milk substitute, too. I'm the worst. But soy milk is not actually much better than industrialized dairy—and for some of the same basic reasons.

Soy can offer some nice benefits: it lowers cholesterol, it's a great source of vegetarian protein, and in some clinical trials, it has helped to regulate hormones. But there are two big problems with it. The first is that soy contains phytoestrogens, which are compounds that are structurally similar to human estrogens and behave in the body like its own natural hormones. Phytoestrogens have been shown to be beneficial in cases where a lack of natural estrogen would lead to health problems. But they've also been shown to be harmful when there is no hormone imbalance.

Women with too much testosterone often suffer from frequent headaches or migraines, terrible PMS, or missing their period often (if you have these symptoms, check in with your doctor). For these women, soy may help with their symptoms and their skin. But obviously hormone balance is a sensitive thing, so for most women, I believe it's best to avoid soy.

The second issue with soy is that, like dairy, it is a very industrialized crop. Almost all of the soy grown in the United States is genetically modified, heavily sprayed with pesticides, and synthetically altered for use in food products. In addition, this industrialized soy is an extremely overused ingredient in the American food system. Like sugar—which you expect to find in a cookie, but probably not in a cracker or your tomato sauce—soy isn't just in veggie burgers and tofu, it's also being slipped into much of what you're eating without your even knowing it: most restaurant food, nut butters, dressings and mayonnaise, canned broth, canned soup, canned tuna, baked goods, cereal, cookies, crackers, and even your baby's formula. If you do find that soy works for you, please don't ignore the ingredient list and opt for an organic source.

Better yet, start buying delicious nut milks and skip this whole issue. Save your soy intake for tempeh, tofu, and miso. If you buy nut milk, be sure to look for sugar-free versions. You can also make your own nut milk, and you will be feeding your body and skin fresh nutrients. And it's a lot easier than you would think—check out the box below!

DIY Nut Milk

1 cup raw organic almonds (or brazil nuts or cashews)

3½ cups water

1 tablespoon honey or maple syrup

Sea salt to taste

Cinnamon and turmeric (optional)

1. Soak the raw almonds (or brazil nuts or cashews) overnight.
2. Drain and rinse the almonds and add to a blender with fresh water and blend until smooth.
3. Pour it through a fine strainer or cheesecloth to separate

out all the solids (use this pulp for a DIY skin-care project or freeze it for use later).

4. Now, add the honey or maple syrup, a small pinch of sea salt, and a pinch of cinnamon and turmeric (both optional) and either stir really well or pour back into the blender for another round.

5. Use it wherever you would use milk or soy milk! It will store in the fridge for about a week, but it's most fresh and delicious during the first few days.

That Fried Chinese Food You Eat "Once in a While"

Believe me, this one breaks my heart more than you can imagine. I love my fried food. Fried veggies in particular can be so ridiculously satisfying, and they feel like the lesser of many evils when it comes to ordering in or dining out. The problem is that you're probably eating it more than every once in a while, and fried food does not contain the kinds of fats you want to be feeding your body.

To begin with, restaurants are not frying food in healthy, organic oils. They are using cheap, low-quality junk oils (like soy, which we just talked about) that do not have the right proportions of essential fatty acids. Plus, when you heat any oil hot enough to fry something, it breaks down the molecules in the oil and creates free radicals. And of course, that wreaks havoc not just with your skin but inside your body, too.

Let's talk about what happens in a commercial fryer. A restaurant fries food in the same super-hot oil over and over again. This causes two things: oxidation and hydrogenation.

In oxidation, the fat breaks down, loses its natural antioxidants, and starts to form free radicals. Hydrogenation causes the fat to change into an ultra-saturated fat, or a trans fat. Our bodies are completely incapable of recognizing trans fats as anything real or natural (because they're not), so we respond with an inflammatory response, as if we are fighting an invader. And we kind of are.

Since the essential fatty acids are crucial to beautiful skin, and you need them in a balanced proportion, you should keep away from commercially fried food. When you really have a craving, make it yourself. Use butter or an organic vegetable oil. You will naturally use a lot less than a restaurant does, but try to cook your food in a small layer of frying oil, not enough to completely submerge it. If you own a deep fryer, I'm sorry, but I'm going to need you to throw it out. And be aware of how much salt you are adding as well, since fried food and lots of salt tend to go together, and the added salt will dehydrate your skin and body.

That Food That Came in a Wrapper

Packaged foods are a super-bad habit for approximately thirty different reasons. Turn that wrapper over. See those ingredients? Guess how many are good for your skin? Guess how many of them clog your pores, cause inflammation and digestive upset, and slow your body down?

I know we already talked about processed foods, but this is slightly different. This is that "healthy" bar you eat every morning, that low-calorie pack you had for dessert, that "high-fiber fortified" cereal you enjoyed two bowls of, those "organic veggie" puffs/sticks/crackers you snacked on, and anything else that comes packaged but because you bought it at Whole Foods or Trader Joe's you think it's okay. Unless you are eating an organic, non-GMO, whole-food bar (with three ingredients that are real foods) because you are about to have or just had the workout of your life, you are hurting yourself and your skin. You are hitting your body with processed sugar, processed fat, processed protein, processed dairy, synthetic flavor (um, yeah, that "natural flavor" is synthetic flavor with a marketing spin), fake coloring, sodium, and preservatives that are sometimes worse than what's in your skin-care products. I mean, if you wrote out a list of all the things no one should ever eat again, it would probably be the ingredient list on most packaged foods, even the healthy ones. And even when they're not bad, they're also just not fresh. I call them dead ingredients. That's really how you should think of them. Once something is packaged, it's a product, not so much a food.

The more you eat these ingredients, the more you will break out and the more you will have depleted skin that looks unhealthy and aged. Every time you consume this type of food, you work against all of the whole, nutrient-dense foods you've given your body, because it takes your body so much work and energy to figure out what to do with all of the dead ingredients, how to process them, and how to get rid of them, fast.

It can be really, really hard to stay away from packaged food, especially because of how busy most of us are these days. Read the ingredient list and look for the more natural alternative (the one with lots of proof that the company is at least paying attention to their ingredients—things like certifications and an explanation of how the product is made), but try to limit your packaged food intake as much as possible.

That Meat You Had at the Airport/Barbecue/Deli

Maybe you discovered by keeping your food journal that you feel great when you eat meat. Hallelujah, right?! But now, just when you thought you could eat all the meat you wanted without feeling guilty, I'm pulling the rug out from under you. I know, so rude!

The science is very clear about meat. If you eat it once or twice a week, you are golden. If you are eating it more often, but it is grass-fed, free-range meat from a trusted farmer who has been doing things the traditional way for generations, that is just great. Really.

But if you make exceptions every other day, every day, or multiple times a day, then you are consuming antibiotics and hormones that were fed to an animal that weighs almost ten times as much as you. All of that garbage is now going into your body. And as we've discussed, you'd better believe it's going to affect the precious balance of your hormones and good bacteria in your gut, not to mention your immune system, which makes your skin suffer, too.

That Third Portion of Anything You've Had Today

I know that overeating is a very touchy subject for many of us. But the fact of the matter is that when you eat, your body becomes just very slightly inflamed. It's negligible and obviously has only a minimal effect; after all, *not* eating is not an option.

But think about the idea that when you eat a normal portion of healthy food, you get just a little inflamed and your body turns its attention toward digestion for a brief moment. Now imagine if you eat something that's hard to digest, devoid of helpful fiber or nutrients, or just downright foreign (aka, processed and synthetic). Now imagine you have a huge breakfast, then you eat a snack midmorning, then a quick lunch, a midafternoon snack, you graze at home before dinner, then you have dinner, then you grab a midnight snack, and the whole day is sprinkled with packaged or nutrient-depleted foods. This is most definitely 100 percent how most people actually eat, and it is just too taxing on your system. It stops your body from being able to take care of itself and provide you with energy, and, of course, that means it also stalls how much of your body's energy can be used to give you good skin and good health in general. It makes you slightly inflamed all the time. You're working against yourself when you are eating a lot, and all of the time.

The first thing most of us should do is to get rid of the entire idea of "five small meals a day." Or the idea that you need a snack between every meal in order to "keep your metabolism going." That is a specialty concept. If you are a triathlete or a breast-feeding mother or a yoga instructor teaching three classes a day, you can maybe have lots of small meals throughout the day and be at your optimal health. But most of us do not have specialized bodies with specialized needs, we have everyday bodies so we need everyday advice.

When an average person tries to follow this kind of specialized recommendation, to eat "five small meals a day" for optimal metabolism, let's be honest, the meals will not be small. The average person doesn't have a triathlete's daily life or daily priorities—and she's definitely not burning the kind of calories a triathlete is burning. With an average person's calorie expenditure, five small meals a day should look something like this: a boiled egg, some carrots and celery, a small salad, an apple, a piece of fish with asparagus, one square of dark chocolate. Did I just describe how you eat?

Did I just describe a diet you could follow for more than three days straight, without going bonkers and eating a whole large pizza? There's nothing wrong with you for saying no. It means you're normal! "Five small meals a day" should be wiped from the consciousness of average people living in a culture where food is so abundant it's actually become a health problem.

Sit down at a table and eat controlled portions when you are hungry. When you can't sit down to eat, do not graze. Eat a prepared snack and be done with it. And, yes, preparing snacks is boring, but being prepared is the best way to stop overeating, and overeating is bad for your skin.

Your Culprit Foods

You found something totally random in your food journal, didn't you? A weird one-off food you never would have expected to show up every time you got a stomachache or felt bloated. Maybe it was something you've always assumed was healthy, like eggs or peanut butter or quinoa. Treat yourself as if you are hypersensitive to this food, even if only for a brief time. If you've done an elimination diet and have successfully gone back to eating it, that's great. But remember that different foods can cause problems at different times, and you should regularly check in with yourself. If you don't eat any of the foods on my list of bad habits and you're still experiencing skin issues, then this is the place you need to spend the most time: cutting out foods you have a hunch are the problem for a few weeks at a time, and then gradually reintroducing them.

Keep in mind that if you are hypersensitive to a food and you remove it and then add it back in without any further problem, that doesn't mean you're now free to eat a ton of it and never worry again. For some reason, your body can become overwhelmed and stop processing it correctly. You are slightly egg intolerant, or peanut butter intolerant, or quinoa intolerant. No big deal. Find alternatives as often as you can, and always eat a variety of foods to keep your body in the practice of receiving and metabolizing different types of nutrients.

Alcohol

Alcohol needs its own section because everyone is obsessed with an ultimate and final answer on alcohol. Are you ready? According to Dr. Frank Lipman at the Eleven Eleven Wellness Center in New York City, the scientific answer is that alcohol basically hits your body like liquid sugar. Aside from being addictive and easy to overconsume (impaired judgment, much?), he points out that alcohol can also affect your sleep patterns, anxiety levels, mood, and immune system. And then there's the potential weight gain. Drinking also dehydrates your skin and hair. In the short term, your skin will become bloated and puffy while trying to retain as much water as possible, and in the long run it will become dry and more likely to wrinkle. Your hair will become brittle and more prone to split ends.

So please, do not kid yourself into thinking that you are drinking wine because it's good for you.

You drink alcohol because . . . *life*. You know? And sometimes it's just as important to relax, or deal, or socialize as it is to eat greens. So let yourself off the hook, to a certain extent. To me, alcohol is the ultimate you-are-an-adult food. Don't lie to yourself about it or find excuses. Face the facts about it not being great for you, and then indulge when you want to (just remember to keep sipping that water, too!). If it pops up on your food journal a little more often than you'd like to see it, then cut back. Your skin will brighten, you'll have more energy, and you won't have as many excuses for not cooking meals at home. Plus, you know, fewer embarrassing late-night texts and selfies.

I KNOW I'VE GIVEN you a lot to think about, but don't let yourself get overwhelmed. Do *not* think that, starting from the second you finish this book, you need to flip your whole life on its head. Nothing I've told you should be taken to mean that if you don't do every bit of it, you'll be sick and your skin will be terrible forever. I want you to make decisions in a way that is light and empowered. In other words, you should feel good about your health, not scared and guilty. You should make healthier food choices because they make you feel happy and free. When you start to feel shackled to your routine or controlled by your food, it's time to take a deep breath and a (small) bite of pizza.

CHAPTER 5

THE BEAUTY INDUSTRY IS UGLY

W e're more than halfway through the book and we haven't talked about your skin-care products yet. There are a few reasons for that.

First of all, it's easy to ignore lifestyle and diet and focus instead on searching for that perfect product, even though what we eat and how we live have way more of an impact on skin health than any cream ever could. Products make up a very small piece of the puzzle . . . yet most of us focus our efforts on the hunt for the miracle elixir. So we need to reverse the focus; it's only after you've corrected your habits that you should be thinking about your products and skin-care routine. Otherwise, nothing you do is going to make a lasting difference.

Another reason I've waited to address the issue of products is because it's usually a tough topic for people—nothing makes my clients freak out more than the prospect of changing their skin-care regimen. But why is it so hard for even the healthiest people to question their skin care? Many of my clients have spent a huge part of their adult lives educating themselves about how to eat the "right way." They know to avoid processed foods; they try to buy local and organic; and they try to eat lots of vegetables. But when it comes to their skin care, they use the absolute worst products—and they use a *lot* of them. When I dare to bring up the fact that maybe they aren't using the healthiest products they could be, they are usually not happy to receive this information. Not even a little.

Here's the thing: I know that people don't like to think about what's in the stuff they're putting all over their face and body. And I don't like to scare or upset anyone, so even though I run a company that is 100 percent committed to natural, nontoxic skin care, I'm often shy about discussing how deeply awful the skin-care industry is, and how serious the situation really is. But after starting S.W. Basics four years ago, I have learned more about the industry than I ever thought I would. And I can confirm for you once and for all: the beauty industry is ugly.

MEET THE SUITS WHO MAKE YOUR BEAUTY PRODUCTS

So let's start with the basics: how we got here, why the beauty industry cannot be trusted, and why you should be very, very careful about the products you buy.

First of all, the entire industry is almost completely unregulated. The Food and Drug Administration, or FDA, is technically the agency charged with overseeing cosmetics, fragrance, and personal care. It would and should be responsible for monitoring what goes into all skin-care products sold in the United States. But the FDA's regulatory oversight in this area is pretty limited.[17] Here is a list of what it does and does not control:

- Besides color additives, no product or ingredient requires FDA approval before going to market.
- The FDA does not oversee or set standards for the safety testing of a product or an ingredient before it is used in a product. It only "advises" manufacturers to conduct their own testing.
- The FDA does not register or license cosmetics companies before they open and begin selling products. A company can only voluntarily register.
- The FDA cannot recall a product that is unsafe for public use. (Food: yes; cosmetics: no.) It can "request" that a product be recalled, but the offending company has to *voluntarily* issue the recall.

Why is it that the agency whose job it is to protect the safety of consumers is so limited in what it can actually do to protect the safety of consumers? Let's discuss.

The FDA works very closely with an organization called the Personal Care Products Council (PCPC). The PCPC created and is responsible for funding the Cosmetic Ingredient Review, or CIR, which is the group that tests ingredients for safety. The CIR is wholly responsible for submitting the data to the FDA that is then used to ban or restrict unsafe ingredients.

The PCP defines itself as "the leading national trade association for the cosmetic and personal care products industry . . . for more than 600 member companies, we are the voice on scientific, legal, regulatory, legislative and international issues for the personal care product industry. We are a leading and trusted source of information for and about the industry and a vocal advocate for consumer safety."[18]

Here are some of the "600 member companies" advising the FDA in its decisions and acting on behalf of your safety as the consumer: Avon, L'Oréal, Estée Lauder, Colgate-Palmolive, Coty, Johnson and Johnson, and Procter & Gamble. Also included are the largest third-party manufacturers (meaning, the companies that actually manufacture products on behalf of the companies that own the brand on the label) of personal-care products in the United States, as well as the chemical manufacturers who supply their ingredients.

In 2014, Michael Taylor, the deputy commissioner of the FDA, wrote a public, very strongly worded letter to the PCPC and ICMAD (Independent Cosmetic Manufacturers and Distributors, another organization that represents 700 personal-care companies), reprimanding both groups for trying to further limit the power of the FDA by calling for even softer regulations. According to Taylor's letter (posted on the FDA's Web site[19]), these industry groups had requested the following actions from the U.S. government:

- For Congress to declare a wide range of potentially harmful chemicals as safe for use in cosmetics without a credible scientific basis.
- For the FDA to affirmatively find other cosmetic ingredients "safe," even if the FDA has determined that they pose real and substantial risks to consumers.
- For the FDA to undergo a lengthy, unnecessarily burdensome process before declaring an ingredient

unsafe, delaying actions to protect consumers by removing unsafe chemicals from cosmetics.

- To virtually eliminate the FDA's ability to verify that cosmetic companies have substantiated the safety of their products.
- To remove the FDA's ability to enforce quality control for the safe manufacturing of cosmetics.
- To prevent the FDA from receiving reports of most illnesses and injuries from improperly manufactured or otherwise dangerous cosmetics, as well as adding a provision that would severely undermine the FDA's ability to use the reporting system for its fundamental purpose: to detect signals of harm from cosmetics.
- To strip the FDA of its authority to require cosmetic companies to register annually with them, thereby reducing the agency's ability to know who is making cosmetic products to sell and what those products are.
- For the U.S. government to stop regulation of the cosmetics industry completely.

The PCPC is lobbying for a host of legal loopholes when it comes to consumer safety. If it gets its way, baby shampoo will be allowed to cause skin and eye irritation; it can be considered unsafe only if it causes blindness or permanent scarring. Adult hair care will be allowed to make your hair fall out; it can be banned only if the hair doesn't grow back. Moisturizer will be allowed to cause blistering and to burn your skin; it just can't permanently disfigure you. And allergic reactions to makeup will be allowed as long as your life is not threatened.

So what *can* the FDA do? If the FDA believes that a company is selling banned or spoiled ingredients (adulteration) or is lying (misbranding), it will take action, in the form of warning letters that threaten legal ramification. You can find the warning letters from the past decade on the FDA's Web site. The last one sent was in 2012. To ensure companies are not using adulterated ingredients, they conduct random and mandatory audits. I'm going to go out on a limb here and say that, in order to do audits, the FDA would need at least to *know* about all the companies that are in business.

I launched my first handmade products online and at craft markets in 2009. Now, we hire third-party manufacturing facilities to make the products, and we sell them directly to our customers online and in stores. Guess how many regulators or authorities have knocked on our door in the entire span of the company's history? Zero. In fact, we've had manufacturers (and lawyers) reassure us that the "wait list" is too long and that the auditors are too busy worrying about food companies. "Don't worry," we've been told over and over, "they'll never even get to skin care." I know lots of companies love this (especially those in the PCPC), but you need to remember that it means the safety of your beauty cabinet was entirely decided by the people who made the products, not by scientists, doctors, or Uncle Sam.

I don't want to get preachy here—I firmly believe in your freedom to make purchasing decisions for yourself, your family, and your home—but wouldn't it be nice if that decision was an informed, educated one? It would be helpful if the sole government organization standing between your skin and potentially toxic chemicals was not getting its information from the corporations who make and sell those chemicals. Why can't the FDA go to multiple, industry-independent chemical-reporting agencies for their data? And why can't they provide us with that information?

There are, in fact, other agencies, and they have a lot of research. You may have heard of some of them, like the Environmental Working Group or the Campaign for Safe Cosmetics. These organizations have shown that *thousands* of chemicals that have not been banned in the United States (but many of which have been banned in other countries) are unsafe. They have massive databases filled with research about almost all of the ingredients in our cosmetics. And it's not pretty. It includes statistics linking many common skin-care and cosmetics chemicals to hormone disruption in animals in the wild, low sperm count and infertility in men, respiratory illnesses like asthma, the development of superbugs that resist drugs and cause disease, and, as you probably guessed, cancer. Oh, and that's besides the normal stuff like skin rashes, allergic reactions, contact dermatitis, and many other external ailments.

This lack of reliable information also means that misbranding—where the FDA should actually have some real authority—is relatively common. Most of the claims on product labels—including *natural, organic, hypoallergenic,* and, yes, *anti-aging*—are ultimately just marketing words. For example, a product can be legally labeled as "natural" and contain up to 30 percent synthetic ingredients. Even certified organic products do not need to be 100 percent organic. The FDA tried to clamp down on the use of the word *hypoallergenic* as far back as 1975, saying that companies could not make the claim if they couldn't provide scientific evidence proving that the product caused fewer adverse reactions than their alternatives. Clinique and Almay sued. Eventually, they won.[20] Now, forty years later, any product can be marked with the word *hypoallergenic*. It holds no meaning whatsoever.

So not only do we not know how safe an ingredient is, we also know very little about whether or not the label on a product is accurate. In addition, companies aren't required to list every ingredient on a product label, so labels can be extremely vague—sometimes neglecting to list certain ingredients altogether.

Many of the people I talk to are shocked by this information—they still don't believe that the chemicals in their skin-care products are as much of a problem as the chemicals in their food. There's a widespread attitude that the things we put *on* our bodies don't affect our health as much as what we put *inside* of our bodies. But you'd better believe that beauty products and cosmetics penetrate your skin and get inside of your body, too. When you apply a cream and it disappears into your skin, that's exactly what it's doing—going *into* your skin and traveling straight to your bloodstream. On top of absorbing chemicals, you are also inhaling them and sometimes eating them (like in your lip balm and toothpaste).

Some progress is currently being made to improve the standards in the beauty industry, though the pace is incredibly slow. The Safe Cosmetics and Personal Care Products Act—which has still not passed—would require cosmetics companies to disclose the use of any chemicals known to cause cancer, birth defects, or other reproductive harm (at the time this book went to press, the only state to adopt the measure was California). Plastic microbeads used in many exfoliants are slowly being banned state by state. So the PCPC hasn't won entirely. But I can tell you from experience that many manufacturers believe that "natural" skin care is only a trend, that it won't have a lasting impact, and that eventually all products will be made from synthetic ingredients.

I would suggest that if your goal is to have good skin, you first need to be aware of exactly what you are putting on it every single day.

THE WORST INGREDIENTS EVER

The following list of chemicals commonly found in cosmetics and personal-care products are the ones that I believe are the worst offenders of all. You'll see I've organized this list by the actual names of the chemicals—not the names you will find listed on your cosmetics labels. So without further ado, I present to you the Worst Ingredients Ever, where they are found, what they can do to you, and the aliases they may be hiding under.

Formaldehyde and Formaldehyde-Releasing Preservatives

Where it is: Nail polish, eyelash glue, hair gel, color cosmetics, and sometimes shampoo. Used as a preservative in a lot of products.

What it does: When inhaled as a gas, formaldehyde causes bronchitis and pneumonia. Also causes contact dermatitis and migraines. Formally classified as carcinogenic to humans.

Check the label for: DMDM hydantoin; diazolidinyl urea; imidazolidinyl urea; and quaternium-15; sodium hydroxymethylglycinate; 2-bromo-2-nitropropane-1, 3-diol.

Plastic and Plasticizers

Where it is: Shampoo and conditioner, as well as a wide array of other beauty products. Gives products a more uniform consistency and makes them more pourable.

What it does: Affects your hormones; is linked to cancer. Plastic microbeads soak up toxins and, when they get into our water supply, disrupt the digestion of small fish and other marine animals that are then eaten by larger fish, which pollutes the entire food chain.

Check the label for: Polyethylene, polythene, PE, phthalates.

Petroleum

Where it is: Moisturizers and lip balms. Petroleum traps water in your skin; some derivatives are used as preservatives.

What it does: Contaminated by known carcinogens, petroleum is linked to kidney and liver abnormality, and it damages cell membranes. Its "trapping" ability also clogs your pores and prevents your skin from getting oxygen.

Check the label for: Petroleum oil, petroleum jelly, petrolatum, mineral oil, mineral jelly, liquid paraffin. Derivatives include propylene glycol, propanediol, and isopropyl alcohol.

Asbestos

Where it is: Powdered makeup and deodorant. Also in baby powder.

What it does: A well-known carcinogen, asbestos is linked to lung cancer when inhaled.

Check the label for: Talc. Asbestos isn't itself an ingredient in skin care, but it is a common contaminant of talc, which is used because it absorbs excess oil from the skin and keeps you dry.[21] Asbestos coexists with talc in nature, and virtually no talc that comes into the United States is tested for asbestos contamination. Also called talcum powder and hydrous magnesium silicate.

Lead

Where it is: Hair dye and lipstick. Contaminates minerals that are used to color products; sometimes used as a colorant itself.

What it does: Lead is a neurotoxin that affects the brain, and a confirmed carcinogen. Lead can build up in the body and develop into lead poisoning, which causes seizures, disrupts child development, and can even be fatal.

Check the label for: Lead acetate.

Coal Tar

Where it is: Hair dye, shampoos (acts as an antidandruff agent). Often used in cosmetics to denature alcohol (a chemical process used to make alcohol undrinkable).

What it does: Coal tar causes skin sensitivity, photosensitivity, and is carcinogenic.

Check the label for: Surprisingly, it's usually just called "coal tar."

THIS LIST OF THE top offenders, sadly, is just the tip of the iceberg—there are so many dangerous chemicals in the products you probably use every day, I could write a whole other book on that topic alone. And because this problem is so big and so pervasive, the answer isn't as easy as just scanning the labels for a few ingredients to avoid (although you should always avoid the ingredients listed above). The solution is to learn how to read a product label.

HOW TO READ A PRODUCT LABEL

Most beauty products are formulated almost entirely of questionable synthetic ingredients. Many of us have gotten into the habit of scrutinizing our food labels and studiously reading the ingredient list on every jar of pasta sauce, package of cookies, or box of cereal we pick up at the store. I want you to do the same thing with your beauty products. You have to learn to differentiate between a synthetic ingredient and a natural one, and then you have to know a little bit about the natural ones, too.

DECODING
the SYMBOLS

The product has been Certified Organic by the USDA, which means it contains at least 95 percent certified organic agricultural ingredients and was produced in a certified organic manufacturing facility.

EcoCert is an organic certification agency started in Europe. Their organic standards meet those of the USDA.

This means the product has been certified free of all animal testing by an international organization called Leaping Bunny.

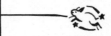

This logo is similar to the Leaping Bunny, but the certifying agency is People for the Ethical Treatment of Animals (PETA).

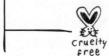

This is basically the expiration date of a personal care product. It tells you how long, in months, that a product will take to go bad after it is first opened.

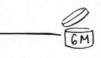

This one looks crazy, but it just means that there is legally required information printed somewhere other than the primary packaging (most often, that's the outer box). Basically it means, "Look inside for more information."

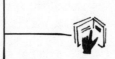

"Naturalwashing" Is the New Greenwashing
A good rule of thumb is to stay away from products that call out one "natural" ingredient on the front label: "shea butter shampoo," "argan oil treatment," "avocado mask"— chances are, that one ingredient is the only natural one it contains, and sometimes even *that* ingredient is a synthetic version of the original. This is just a form of greenwashing.[22]

First, let's talk about INCI, which stands for International Nomenclature of Cosmetic Ingredients. It is the worldwide standard for writing ingredients so they are understood everywhere. When a product uses INCI "language" to list its ingredients, it can look like a confusing list of chemicals. But it's actually either the full, proper chemical name, or it's a natural ingredient written in Latin. So a paraben will be "Methylparaben," and water will be "Aqua." Shea butter will be "Butyrospermum Parkii (Shea) Butter" and oat bran will be "Avena Sativa (Oat) Bran," but sodium laureth sulfate will still just be "Sodium Laureth Sulfate." It might seem intimidating to discern, but don't be afraid of INCI lists. Companies that use this language aren't necessarily trying to hide things from you; they may just be exporting their products to other countries. Sometimes you will see lists that contain the INCI name as well as the common name in parentheses, such as "Sodium Chloride (Sea Salt/Sel de Mer)." In this case, the manufacturer is actually trying to clarify their ingredients for you. Since salt isn't a plant ingredient, INCI requires that the company write out the scientific name for salt, which, in this case, is its chemical name. This type of labeling is a positive trend, because it indicates that manufacturers know you are reading labels—and they want you to be able to understand the words you find there.

≡LOOKING at LABELS≡

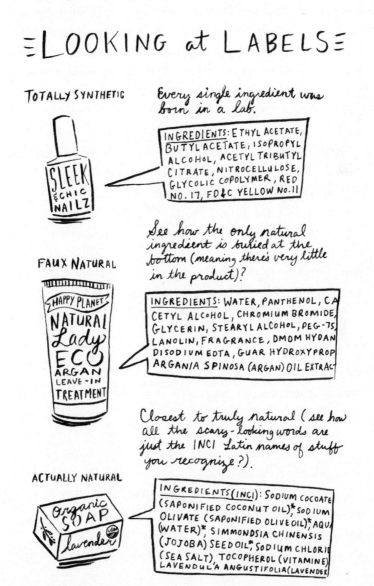

TOTALLY SYNTHETIC

Every single ingredient was born in a lab.

SLEEK & CHIC NAILZ

INGREDIENTS: ETHYL ACETATE, BUTYL ACETATE, ISOPROPYL ALCOHOL, ACETYL TRIBUTYL CITRATE, NITROCELLULOSE, GLYCOLIC COPOLYMER, RED NO. 17, FD&C YELLOW NO. 11

FAUX NATURAL

See how the only natural ingredient is buried at the bottom (meaning there's very little in the product)?

HAPPY PLANET NATURAL Lady ECO ARGAN LEAVE-IN TREATMENT

INGREDIENTS: WATER, PANTHENOL, CA CETYL ALCOHOL, CHROMIUM BROMIDE, GLYCERIN, STEARYL ALCOHOL, PEG-75 LANOLIN, FRAGRANCE, DMDM HYDAN DISODIUM EDTA, GUAR HYDROXYPROP ARGANIA SPINOSA (ARGAN) OIL EXTRAC

ACTUALLY NATURAL

Closest to truly natural (see how all the scary-looking words are just the INCI Latin names of stuff you recognize?).

Organic SOAP lavender

INGREDIENTS(INCI): SODIUM COCOATE (SAPONIFIED COCONUT OIL)*, SODIUM OLIVATE (SAPONIFIED OLIVE OIL)*, AQU (WATER)*, SIMMONDSIA CHINENSIS (JOJOBA) SEED OIL*, SODIUM CHLORI (SEA SALT), TOCOPHEROL (VITAMIN E) LAVENDULA ANGUSTIFOLIA (LAVENDER

On the other hand, if you find something like: "Sodium Levulinate (from Corn)," or "Potassium Sorbate (Food-Grade Preservative)," or "Sodium Lauroyl Methyl Isethionate (Derived from Coconut)," you should be wary. When the translation is not a literal translation—like, "Sodium Chloride (Sea Salt)"—it's because marketing language has come into play. The manufacturer wants you to see that a now-synthetic ingredient was once coconut or corn. They're attempting to convince you that the product is in some way "natural" because its ingredients were found in nature before they were processed into something else. It's just like food packaging changing "artificial flavors" to "natural flavors." There is no difference. These are all synthetic ingredients with convenient explanations.

And to be clear, I don't think all food-derived ingredients are life-threatening. I'm not trying to boss you into boycotting the beauty aisle; I am saying you need to read product labels, understand what the words mean, and then make decisions for yourself about where and when to cut back.

And when in doubt, do some research.

WHY GO NATURAL?

This is a question that I get a lot. If you remain unconvinced that what is in your skin care matters after reading about the lack of regulation, testing, or label honesty in this industry . . . I now present you with the top three excuses I hear from people all the time, and my responses to them. (As if you needed three more reasons to go natural.)

But chemicals are everywhere! It doesn't matter what I do, I am going to be exposed to them . . . Why make myself crazy?

Just because chemicals are everywhere and unavoidable does not mean you should also literally bathe yourself in them. That's like saying that pollution is horrible and we can't do anything about it, so why even bother taking a breath of fresh, clean air when you get the chance. Your skin needs as many breaks as it can get from the chemicals.

Isn't it possible that the natural stuff could also make me break out?
It is possible that anything could make you break out. In the meantime, while no one has ever found coconut oil in a tumor, they have found parabens in tumors. Being exposed to too much aloe has never given someone cancer, but being exposed to too much coal tar has.

I use some "toxic" products but feel totally fine. Maybe those ingredients just don't affect me?
Just because you aren't experiencing noticeable symptoms right this very moment doesn't mean the health effects of dangerous products are nonexistent. That is what makes them so scary. You may have a mild symptom that you overlook, or you may have a cluster of seemingly unrelated symptoms that you would never connect to your beauty routine. Chemicals in some hair dyes have been linked to asthma. If you are experiencing asthma symptoms and you have had a standing appointment at the salon every few months for the past twenty years to get your hair dyed, would you necessarily notice a connection between the two? Just because you haven't recognized the connection doesn't mean it's not there.

Whole, natural ingredients are exactly what they sound like: ingredients that come directly from nature, meaning a plant (and sometimes an animal—not that I'm into that, but animals are part of nature). They may require some processing in order to exist, like in the case of oils and hydrosols (think rosewater and witch hazel), but they were not created by chemistry. In the 1980s, the Federal Trade Commission defined a "natural ingredient" as one that could contain no synthetic or artificial components, and could not have been processed beyond what someone could do in their kitchen.[23] It is in this spirit that I refer to natural ingredients.

Now that you're done arguing with me, it's time for the really fun part.

CHAPTER 6

THE SKIN CLEANSE

Welcome to the guts of this book. This is where you and I work some magic.

At this point, you've cleaned up your diet, or at least you're working on it. You know so much about the cosmetics industry and what your beloved products really consist of that you've already purged your bathroom cabinet of the worst offenders. As far as I'm concerned, you're already a whole new person.

In many plans or programs, this would be the point at which I'd tell you that you know everything you need to know to live a healthy lifestyle and to get that beautiful, glowing skin you've always dreamed about. Just follow all of my instructions with 100 percent precision and never look at a French fry ever again. Bye-bye and good luck!

That's how I felt after I completed nutrition school. Like I had all the information, all of the right rules to follow, but somehow it wasn't adding up. I was doing everything right: eating super-clean, exercising every day, and using natural products. But still I struggled with acne, folliculitis, and an itchy scalp.

Actually, "struggling" is putting it lightly. I was losing it. I was so, so, so frustrated. My face was inflamed. My legs were itching constantly. Every morning I woke up with bloody sheets after clawing at my legs in my sleep. I was a disaster. I had a hunch that something in my products was making my skin freak out, so I tried a million different brands. Still, nothing helped.

So I gave up. I stopped using everything. Every single product. I'm talking I went completely cold turkey. I washed with water only. No soap, no body wash, no shampoo. No makeup. No moisturizer. Nothing. The only personal-care products I continued using were toothpaste and deodorant.

And that's when everything got better—and I really mean *everything*.

Let me take a step back. If it were up to the personal-care industry, your daily routine would look something like this: wake up, shower with shampoo, conditioner, body wash, shaving cream; brush teeth, floss, use mouthwash; wash face, apply astringent, serum, moisturizer, primer, sunscreen, and bronzer. Then deodorant. Oh, and this is all before you even start thinking about makeup. And perfume. Throughout the day, you would turn to your face-blotting sheets, face spritzer, hand sanitizer, hand soap, and hand cream. At night, maybe you shower again, but this time, you apply a deep conditioner first (because you can never condition enough, right?). You remove your makeup, exfoliate (sometimes with a really expensive piece of equipment), and then apply eighteen different serums or lotions because there is one for your eyes, one for your T-zone, one for your neck, one for your elbows and knees, one for your legs, and one for your feet. On the weekends, this routine is twice as long. (It's a wonder day spas are still in business!)

Here's what those companies would never want you to do: wake up, brush teeth, splash water on face, apply a natural moisturizer (maybe even just some coconut oil or olive oil from your pantry), use deodorant, and apply mascara. Go out. Come home. Quickly clean face and mascara off with more oil from your kitchen, wash hair with shampoo. Go to bed. Condition hair only on weekends, use a face cleanser once a week, and exfoliate once a month. Make a homemade face mask once in a blue moon for fun or for furious skin (a breakout; a sunburn; or dry, chapped skin from freezing weather).

The routine I just described is exactly my routine. It is the one and only routine I have ever found that soothes my skin and keeps my terrible skin freak-outs away. You know how when you do an elimination diet and offer your body a chance to detox, you usually see quick and dramatic changes (you do know this, because you have done it, yes?)? Well, guess what—after I quit my former skin-care habits cold turkey and detoxed from my products, my skin responded immediately, enthusiastically, and happily. Since then, I've put every client I've ever had on a version of this routine—even if it's only for a few days—and it has made a huge difference every time.

I'm not saying that lifestyle and diet aren't important. For long-term relief of skin issues and lasting health, especially, the way you choose to eat and to live are paramount. But when it comes to the skin ailments that nag you from day to day, quitting your products is how you get better. Period.

BEFORE THE CLEANSE

Step 1: Start with a Product Journal

If the idea of spending a panicked Saturday on the floor of your bathroom reading every label in your medicine cabinet and looking up each ingredient on the Environmental Working Group's Skin Deep database doesn't really excite you—and I can't imagine why it wouldn't—then the best way to start rethinking your skin-care routine is by taking a look at the products you use as a whole. You can do this by keeping a product journal.

A product journal is exactly like a food journal, but instead of meticulously recording what you ingest, you record what you put on your body. It'll be slightly easier to keep track of than your food, but equally enlightening. No one ever thinks to keep a product journal. Face it: we love buying skin care—there are probably over two dozen products in your cabinet right now—and we also love to change up what we're using constantly. It's so fun and really can make you feel awesome. But this means you're adding more and more products to your cabinet and using them all without really thinking about whether or not you need to use them. Truly, when was the last time you reconsidered your entire routine? When you were sixteen? I thought so. You know when most women do it for the second time? When they're pregnant. And that's about it. But at other points in your life you struggle with how to get your skin right, or normal, or just not so unpredictable, dammit, without considering that maybe your products are part of the problem.

Think of it this way: let's say you use ten products on your face every day—face wash, day cream, foundation, powder, blush, makeup remover, different face wash, eye cream, serum, and spot treatment. And let's say on top of that, five of those are the same every day, but five of them you rotate out because you like to change it up. And lastly, let's say each of those products has a list of ten ingredients (and please, I'm being incredibly conservative with that number; the list of ingredients for each is probably much, much longer!).

What if you're sensitive to just one of the ten ingredients in one of the ten products you use? What if something super-simple, and possibly even natural, like rosemary, triggers some kind of a reaction? That means you will break out or have irritated skin every single day and have absolutely no idea what's causing it, because you are putting 100 ingredients on your face every day. Worse, you might increase that number by slathering on even more products in the belief that there's something wrong with you and you just aren't using the right stuff.

This is where a product journal is priceless. Just like with your food, taking note of every product you use each day will blow you away. First of all, you'll instantly realize what a junkie you are. You'll start to think about how much extra time you would have to sleep or make counter 'kraut if you didn't spend it on your fifteen-step routine. But then you'll get brave enough to experiment with cutting back, and that's when you'll find the problem products.

And for all of you one-step ladies out there, don't scoff at the product journal and think it won't help you. Unless you have perfect skin (in which case you should go read something by Ms. Paltrow), then there is always something to discover by taking a look at your routine. Just because you roll out of bed each day and do nothing more than coat yourself from head to toe with coconut oil doesn't mean you have found your perfect product. If you are seeing skin issues, then take a fresh look at your routine—no matter how simple it is. Although, the simpler it is, the easier it'll be to spot the problem.

Just take note, for three to seven days, of what products you use and when. You don't need to keep track of all the extras (mood, digestion, sleep, headaches, and that kind of stuff) like you did in your food journal. But you should continue to pay close attention to the state of your skin at various times of the day. Check in more often than you did during your food journal. I recommend that every time you go to the bathroom you give yourself a good once-over in the mirror. Are you dry in the morning but oily at night? Do you get itchy after a shower?

And, like with the food journal, look for combinations and unlikely coincidences. Oh, wait, you just realized you break out every time you apply foundation but not when you skip it on the weekends? Every time you use your new face wash you seem to get chapped lips? That fancy $300 shampoo appeared in your shower around the same time as your back acne? Those are not coincidences.

Here are a few other things to consider as you begin your product journal:

- Every product matters, even if you think it doesn't. This includes hand soap, dish soap, hand sanitizer, lip balm, deodorant. If it touches your skin, write it down.
- If you have a pet or spend time with someone else's, keep track of that, too. Even if you're not full-blown allergic, you could have a very slight allergy, and the cuddles could be the thing making you itchy.

- How frequently you're using the same product may affect how well it's working. Pay attention to the products you use every day versus the ones you use only every so often so that you can look for patterns later.
- Your exercise habits, plus how you deal with your skin after you exercise, will matter. Take note of times you were unable to shower, forgot to wash your face, or changed what you used to clean your skin because you were at the gym.
- The same is true for being away from home in general. If you leave town and use hotel amenities, a friend's products, your parents' amenities, or you quickly grab travel sizes at the store, write this down. Take note that you are traveling, which also can be hard on some people's skin even if you pack all of your own products.
- Pay attention to your laundry detergent, especially if you recently changed it or change it while journaling.
- Also think about how much dirt comes into contact with your skin. Mark down when you wash your pillowcases and bedsheets, and when you get sweaty and can't change your clothing (in other words, if the sweat dries and you are in the same clothes, write this down and watch for symptoms).
- Try to pay attention to how much you pick at your skin (or touch it other than when you're washing it). Picking at your face has a trifecta of negative effects: it transfers bacteria from your hands to your face (and not the good kind), it fills your pores with more oil from your hands, and it stops blemishes from healing by reopening the wounds.
- Be very honest with yourself about how much makeup you put on, how often you remove it, and with what.

Before you get started, here's a sample two-day product journal from another one of my amazing, fearless clients. Note that she doesn't go into a lot of detail, but is meticulous about tracking every single personal-care item that she comes into contact with each day.

DAY ONE:

(One new breakout)

Trader Joe's tea tree face wash

Dove soap

Paul Mitchell tea tree shampoo

Yes to Carrots conditioner

Colgate Total toothpaste

Scope mouthwash

Secret deodorant

Laura Mercier foundation powder

Tarte Blush

Tarte Eyeliner

Maybelline Great Lash mascara

Clinique makeup remover

Proactiv mask

Proactiv lotion

DAY TWO:

(The breakout is bigger and face feels a little sensitive)

Trader Joe's tea tree face wash

Proactiv scrub

Dove soap

Paul Mitchell tea tree shampoo

Yes to Carrots conditioner

Colgate Total toothpaste

Scope mouthwash

Nivea Extended Moisture lotion

Secret deodorant

Laura Mercier foundation powder

Sephora eye shadow

Maybelline Great Lash mascara

Nail polish remover

Clinique makeup remover

Proactiv mask

Proactiv lotion

I actually worked with this client for a few months, and she had severe breakouts the whole time—the kind that are red and irritated and take a long time to go away. It took the product journal for her to realize she just has very sensitive skin. It wasn't one product giving her issues, it was almost all of them. She cut back to using only a natural, gentle soap for one day and stopped breaking out. *One* day. She made dietary tweaks that helped her skin continue to improve over time, but the relief from cutting out products happened overnight.

The product journal is mostly meant to show you how many beauty products you're actually using. But if you pay close attention while you do it, you'll start to notice irritated skin right after you use a problem product. If you wake up with a blemish, it may be linked to a product you used the day before. If you are itchy, take a look at the product in the journal closest to the time you became itchy; it basically needs enough time to dry on your skin before you have this type of reaction. The same is true for really dry skin; a bad product will make you dry almost instantly. Oily skin means your products are too harsh; your skin is producing oil to protect itself. It also means your beloved moisturizer isn't working. Body breakouts are most likely the result of your shampoo, conditioner, or body wash. Chronically chapped, irritated lips can come from your lip products but also from your face wash or shampoo. Steady acne usually means you have very sensitive skin, so all of the products in your journal may be causing different blemishes to appear.

I think it's pretty powerful to physically write down the list, but to make it even easier, you can also line up all the products you use in a day on your bathroom sink and take a picture with your phone. Set up a photo album for the days when you're product journaling. Just keeping track is eye-opening in itself, and, if later you start to suspect that one product in particular is aggravating your skin, you'll have a record of which ingredient labels you should take a good hard look at.

Step 2: Think About Your Makeup

I'm not going to try to convince you that you have to switch to a 100 percent natural makeup routine. To be honest, I haven't even made that transition completely myself. I think you should use natural makeup (and I think I should, too), but since I hardly ever wear makeup, I have a really hard time paying forty bucks for a concealer I'll apply maybe once a month. You'll make your own compromises based on your lifestyle, too. So yes, you can keep your makeup. But I am going to have to insist that you keep it fresh, remove it every night, and study that product journal to see how much of it you use.

JUNKIE you

SOBER you

MORNING ROUTINE
- Acne wash + toner
- Anti-wrinkle serum
- leave-in hair treatment
- oil-free moisturizer
- Beachy hair volumizer
- Anti-perspirant
- Floral perfume
- Raspberry Body Butter
- Whitening toothpaste
- foundation, blush, lipstick, etc...

INGREDIENT TALLY: 200

MORNING ROUTINE
- Homemade toothpaste
- Baking Soda Zit Zapper
- Coconut oil after shave
- aloe Sea Salt hair spray
- homemade shea butter moisturizer
- lip balm
- a few splashes of cool water

INGREDIENT TALLY: 20

When was the last time you bought new makeup? Are you still using the same mascara your mom gave you at the holidays that one year? Gross. Makeup does go bad, you know. One of the reasons these products are so problematic in the first place is because they're full of chemicals that extend the shelf life about a thousand times longer than it should be—but they're still not immortal. And just imagine, if that preservative was extending the shelf life of the product by a few years already, by the time it starts to grow mold or bacteria, that stuff is going to be super-nasty. Every single skin condition is exacerbated by spoiled makeup. Virtually all cosmetics have expiration dates on them. Find the date, and if it has come and gone, toss the product. If you've had it so long the expiration date has rubbed off, toss the product. If both of those options don't pan out, you can tell a product has expired if the smell is very strong or the consistency is chunky or thicker than normal. You can always stop by the store and compare what you have to a fresh product. And to save time, just buy the fresh one while you're there.

When it comes to removing your makeup—I get that accidents happen. Everyone has days when they get home from work late and are too exhausted even to remember to wash their face. Days when you're traveling and don't have time to run to the hotel to take off yesterday's makeup before heading to dinner. Nights when you fall asleep on the couch watching a movie and can barely summon the energy to turn off Netflix and walk to the bedroom. And of course, there are those nights where a few cocktails have blurred the edges, and removing makeup isn't at the forefront of your mind when you make it home.

I get it: life happens, and sometimes makeup removal doesn't. But here's the thing: when you wake up the next day with a breakout, you should know that this is why. I would name long-worn makeup as the number one cause of breakouts on skin that is otherwise symptom-free. Think about it: the whole point of makeup is to physically cover up the outermost layer of your skin so that people see the makeup and not you. When you leave your makeup on for a long time, you're letting all those chemicals sit on your face all day and sometimes all night, and when you don't remove it completely, you just keep layering more of it on.

Despite the urban legend you may have heard about the

lady whose eyelashes fell out after she left her mascara on overnight—your eye makeup is actually the least of your worries. If you're going to pick what to focus on and get lazy about, I'd like to urge you to start with your face, which means your foundation, powder, blush, concealer. Take your time removing your makeup. You need to make sure that you really massage your face and wipe it clean. Makeup remover is not going to make you break out, and if yours does, then you shouldn't be using it. For face makeup, you should generally use remover and then also wash your face. The more intense the makeup (think more than two layers, or makeup designed to survive a war), the stronger your cleanser should be. So for example, this is one of the few instances I would recommend using a natural soapy face wash. The foam will help dissolve your makeup so that it rinses off more easily.

If you are pleasantly surprised that your makeup remover wipes everything away in one swipe, please consider what may be in it that allows it to have supernatural powers. Sometimes the compromise is that a little more work = healthier skin. This is especially true with remover, since the most powerful ones are loaded with chemicals and alcohol, and they are going onto (and sometimes into) your eyes, one of the most sensitive parts of your body. Keep in mind that as you wipe away your eye makeup, it, too, is going into your eyes—so don't assume that stinging feeling is a result of the remover. That industrial-strength eyeliner you've had since 2009 that contains coal tar is more likely to be the culprit.

Although you need to give this step some love, taking off your makeup does not need to be an hour-long endeavor. There are definitely great natural makeup removers on the market. Look for an oil-based remover, especially if you wear

waterproof makeup. Even your eye cream or a single ingredient like argan oil can work as a makeup remover. So can a
really rich face moisturizer. And in a pinch, you can use olive
oil and a cotton ball. Here are the other pantry staples I recommend for taking off makeup:

- Olive oil
- Sesame oil (make sure it's not toasted sesame unless you
  want to smell like Chinese food)
- Coconut oil
- Grapeseed oil
- Avocado oil
- Sunflower oil

You can use each of these oils on its own, or you can mix
a few of them together, which will offer even more nutrients
for your skin. And you don't need to worry about washing
them off, just keep wiping until the makeup is gone and the
cotton ball looks clean. Unless you have had on twenty layers
of makeup for a special occasion—in which case, follow it up
with a sudsy cleanser.

I know you're not going to stop wearing makeup. And you
will always have the nights where you would rather die than
take the time to go through the process of taking it off. But
make sure you create some kind of makeup-removal ritual that
is as normal for you as brushing your teeth, and then *stick to
it.* Do it as often as you possibly can. Think of it as letting
your pores breathe again; imagine that, while you sleep, your
skin is basically detoxing. You're pressing the Reset button so
that you wake up fresh the next day. Clean bedtime skin will
solve more of your skin problems than you realize.

Sleep Is a Beauty Product

Have you ever noticed that when you don't sleep well, your skin looks dull and puffy? That is not an illusion; it's a real thing. During sleep, collagen production accelerates. Growth hormones also peak, which helps restore and regenerate your skin cells. In fact, in a 2013 study, better sleep was linked to faster recovery from environmental stressors.[24] Sleeping well helps regulate the production of the stress hormone cortisol throughout the day, and we know that too much cortisol ages us. So turn off the TV, take your makeup off, get in bed, and have sweet dreams about beautiful skin.

Step 3: Check Yourself into Beauty Rehab

Let me be clear: I don't believe there is anything more important for ensuring the long-term health of your skin than this next step. Not one thing will have a greater impact. Not even your diet. You got me? No piece of advice that I have ever given to anyone has ever been as effective as this one. I am not exaggerating when I say that every single client, friend, and skeptic I have convinced to try this step has come back to me in shock and awe. It will change your skin-care life forever.

Here's what we're going to do: since the product journaling showed you to be the true beauty junkie that you are, we're going to break your addiction.

I know that the thought of a single day without your beloved BB Cream may have caused you to slam this book closed and throw it across the room. But that's the amazing thing about a book; it will wait for you to come back, dust off the pages, and try again. If you've forgotten how we got to this point, please go back to Chapter 5 and read it over and over again until you remember why your skin needs a break. Reread Chapter 4 and think about how much better everything gets when you eat less junk. Your skin is the same: put less junk on it, and it will get better.

Some of my clients love the challenge of going completely cold turkey, like I did. The second I suggest the idea of a product break, it's as if they've been waiting for permission to abandon their beauty regimens their whole lives. And some clients actually use few enough products that it doesn't pose that much of a challenge.

Most clients, though, need some convincing, so I lead them a bit more gently through detox—in baby steps. That's why this skin cleanse is customizable! There are three levels: you can start at Level 1 and work your way up to Level 3, or you can go straight to the level that best matches your routine and your goals for your skin. Let's get started.

Level 1: Supplement

Length of time: Three days, more if you love it

Who this is for: Beauty junkies looking for some extra nourishment

This is the level for those of you who feel as if you just can't part with your products or makeup, but you are interested in doing something a little different to get better skin. In Level 1, you don't have to stop using your products; you are just going to add in one or two of the all-natural recipes from Chapter 7 and you'll pick one or two of the ingredients to use on their own.

It's sort of like topical supplementing. Since the ingredients are completely natural, they provide much-needed nutrients for your skin. You should notice smoother, clearer skin within a few days.

Try to choose a recipe from the list below that you think will suit your skin's needs. If you love your moisturizer but are worried your face wash isn't the best, maybe you want to swap in a homemade face wash. If you're thinking of finding a new moisturizer but aren't ready to give yours up, use olive oil after your moisturizer and see if things get better. If you're totally happy with your face-care routine but struggle with body breakouts or rashes, try adding a homemade body scrub. Or if you prefer not to use one of the recipes, select an ingredient or two from the list to mix into your existing products. You can add an exfoliating ingredient to your face wash, an oil to your moisturizer, a "butter" to your mask . . . it won't take much extra time, but you'll definitely feel extra fancy.

Here are some great ingredients to add to your routine. Start by mixing one part ingredient to one part product in your hand or a small bowl, and experiment with more or less as you go:

- Oat flour into your face wash (or try the Reparative Oat-Berry Cookie Exfoliant on page 187 before or after your face wash)
- Olive oil into your moisturizer
- Clay into your shampoo (or make the Hair Mask/ Shampoo on page 201)
- Aloe leaf or juice into your makeup remover
- A cup of sea salt in your bath water (or the Soothing Bath Soak on page 193)
- Honey as a face wash (apply like a mask, then rinse with warm water), then follow with the rest of your routine as normal

You don't need to stick to the same recipes or ingredients every single day. This level is about adding extra nourishment, and that can come from a variety of sources. But if you find that moisturizing with olive oil after you wash your face really does seem to make a huge difference for your skin, you might want to keep it up for a few extra days and see what happens. If a new ingredient helps instantly, it's likely going to help even more over time.

You can stick with Level 1 forever if you want, but I'd say, even if Level 1 is your happy place and you never try Level 2, aim for taking at least one day out of every month to add a high-quality natural ingredient or recipe to your routine. Of course, in my ideal world, you'll love Level 1 so much that you won't be able to wait to try Level 2!

Level 2: Eliminate and Nourish

Length of time: One day

Who this is for: Experiment lovers with nagging skin ailments

In Level 2 you will detox your skin by going sans makeup, sans product for one full day. One day! It's nothing. It will go by in a flash. Pick a day when you plan to lounge around the house, or when you are feeling particularly rebellious. I promise you that if you have to see people, they won't care that you're makeup-free nearly as much as you think they will.

You will not use mascara, blush, eye shadow, or even a "touch of" concealer. Nothing. You will not use your face wash or exfoliant or toner or serum or moisturizer. None of it. You will replace those with the recipes and ingredients in Chapter 7. For Level 2, I recommend choosing from the list below. These are all recipes and ingredients that are super-gentle and will help your skin detoxify and return to its natural pH balance. If you have completed Level 1 successfully and have found something that worked well for you, keep it up and use it on your no-product day.

You don't need to worry about your other personal-care products like shampoo, conditioner, deodorant, and toothpaste—at Level 2, you can stick with your normal non-skin-care products. Though the more products you can skip, the better—so if you don't need to wash your hair that day, maybe you can skip it and eliminate a few more products. If you want to wash your face, use one of the products or ingredients from the list, or use a natural, handmade soap bar or just water (see box below).

How to wash your face with only water

Did you know that you can wash your face without soap? Water is an effective cleanser all on its own. Just make sure you follow a few basic rules:

Make sure your hands are clean. You already wash them or sanitize them a trillion times a day, so chances are they aren't dirty—but do a quick check.

Splash water onto your face, using your clean hands. Aim for ten to twenty splashes. (If this is your first time, I prefer you do twenty. Count them out.)

Use your hands to (gently) rub the water over your face as you go. I do ten splashes where I go up and down with my hands one time per splash.

This whole process should take you thirty to sixty seconds, and then your face will be clean, I swear.

Just like anything else in life, less is more—so I wouldn't recommend trying out more than two or three recipes on your "clean skin day." We're trying to give your skin a break, so don't overwhelm it with seven new homemade products. Pick a toner and an oil, or a body scrub that you can use on your face, too. Wash your face with water and follow it with a spot treatment, or skip everything except a luxurious face mask right before bed.

If you don't want to experiment with recipes, try using a simple, unscented castile soap. Castile soap is saponified olive oil. Though it's gone through a process that makes it less gentle than the oil it came from, it will create suds and the slippery effect that makes you feel really clean. You can use it to wash your hair, your face, and your body. For one day. Follow it up with a full-body coconut oil slather, if you can. Remember, we're just trying to get to a slightly "less is more" place.

Best recipes for Level 2:

- Balancing Oil Cleanser (page 173)
- Brightening Astringent (page 178)
- Deep Sea Hydrating "Strips" (page 185)
- Combination Face and Body Exfoliant (page 191)
- Hair Oil (page 205)

Level 3: Detoxify

Length of time: Three days to two weeks

Who this is for: Courageous truth seekers, the super-sensitive, and *Skin Cleanse* converts

Level 3 is the cold turkey version of beauty rehab. If you're ready to take the plunge, here's what you're going to do: take a break from *all* of your products (makeup, soap, and shampoo included) for at least three days (longer if you can). Forcing you to bravely show your own, naked face to the world for three whole days is the mental-health portion of the program.

The centerpiece of Level 3 is washing both your face and your body with water only. Use a washcloth to get squeaky clean. (Don't worry, I'll still let you use deodorant—although I'd prefer if you use one of the natural deodorant recipes from Chapter 7.) The idea that you *have* to wash with products in order to get clean is marketing hype. Water cleans your skin, and your skin cleans your skin. It doesn't need soap—it needs a break. It needs to breathe.

You will wash your hair with water only, no shampoo, no conditioner. If you absolutely can't skip shampoo, aim to keep your hair care as simple as possible. Maybe you could wash your hair once, with an unscented castile soap. Or follow one of the recipes for a homemade shampoo. By now, you understand what we're going for at this stage, so I'm going to trust you to use your best judgment.

After showering or washing your face, leave your skin alone. You may feel a bit dry. Don't worry, that's normal. Dryness is one of the first ways your skin shows that it's trying to rebalance itself. If you go into a full freak-out over the dryness, use some olive oil. Either way, you are going to allow your skin some space to regulate itself again—something that, because of all the products you've been using, it hasn't had to do in a long time. Each time you wash with only water, your skin should feel a little better. Even the dryness will start to ease over the course of the first three days.

Step 4: Returning to Your Daily Routine

When you are done with your skin cleanse, it will be similar to your coming off an elimination diet—especially if you went all the way to Level 3. But even if you stopped at Level 1, you should be able to make a few subtle discoveries. You will immediately notice that products you thought were helping or that you regarded as everyday staples suddenly cause flare-ups. You will finally be able to see which products, ingredients, or steps in your skin-care routine to abandon.

On the flipside, you'll also notice that the real winners in your regimen will work even better. Your skin will finally respond to them again, but it will also be less dependent on them. It is a win-win. Once you're able to see which products and ingredients are helping you and which are hurting you, go ahead and toss the junk ones. A product elimination is not like a food elimination, where you might be able to take a break from a particular food and then come back to it later. If a product is lousy for your skin, it's just lousy for your skin. Fortunately for you, getting rid of a product means you get to replace it with another and create a whole new beauty cabinet for yourself. Even more fortunately, I've designed a bunch of options for you, from scratch. I know, I'm excited, too.

On that note—let's head to the kitchen.

CHAPTER 7

BE YOUR OWN APOTHECARY

N ow that you've gritted your teeth and scaled back your beauty routine, it's time for the fun part: creating a *new* routine. You've given your skin a much-needed break, but my guess is that you're pretty eager to start using products again. No problem, that's what this chapter is all about! You have come to the right place, friend.

After the skin-care meltdown that led me to discover how insanely helpful it could be to take a cold-turkey beauty break, I gradually discovered a routine that works for me to this day. It's not foolproof, of course. I still get pimples sometimes and itchy skin occasionally, but I never, ever have the devastating skin issues that used to control my life.

I never use products in the morning. Nothing has improved my skin as much as this simple shift. These days, when I'm breaking out from stress or hormones, I use apple cider vinegar to balance my pH. When I get so sweaty I can feel my skin cracking, I exfoliate with sea salt or some almond meal, because who needs plastic microbeads when nature makes perfect exfoliants? I take my makeup off with a combination of sweet almond oil, olive oil, and jojoba oil (none of which clogs your pores), and I treat my hair with shea butter because it helps my split ends *and* my scalp. Through this routine, I have transitioned from horribly problematic skin to happy calm skin almost all of the time.

Fortunately for me, the products I created to take care of my skin became the exact same products that my company, S.W. Basics, now makes and sells, so I have all of the kitchen-cabinet skin-care products I could ever want (though I'm no longer the one making them all by hand!). Even still, I continue to work on my skin-care routine—healthy skin is always a work in progress.

But for now, this should be your goal: fewer products, less money, fewer breakouts, less frustration. Your new skin-care routine will include a few go-to products and some special "treats," all of which are as clean, natural, and packed with as many nutrients as possible. The beauty routine I recommend for my clients is built on just ten ingredients. These kitchen staples—soon to become your skin-care staples—will accomplish everything you could ever want from a beauty product. Once you realize that these natural products can help your skin do what it does best, you'll trust them and will be able to step away from your sudsy, chemical-laden face washes and creams, which are not helping much anyways.

START WITH THESE TEN INGREDIENTS AND YOU'LL NEVER GO BACK

The ingredients that follow make up the foundation of your new beauty routine. You can probably find some of them in your kitchen already, because they're all edible. I suggest you start by playing around with these ingredients before you even get to the recipes. They are incredibly potent on their own, and learning to mix and match them will teach you the basics of being your own little chemist. They're also so bare minimum, it's impossible to be too lazy to try them out.

Fine-grain sea salt is especially great for acne or quick treatments during flare-ups. It can be used on the face or body and cleans deeply, removes dead skin cells, eliminates fluid retention, balances moisture, pulls toxins from pores, and relaxes muscles. Most sea salts are high in magnesium, potassium, calcium, and bromine. The simplest way to use sea salt is to wet your skin, put some salt on your wet hand so it sticks, then pat it gently onto your skin. You can leave it for a few minutes or rinse immediately. Just make sure not to scrub too hard—it is too abrasive by itself.

Apple cider vinegar is the best astringent in nature because it helps to balance your skin's pH, making you both less oily *and* less dry. Plus, it promotes blood circulation and kills bacteria, yeasts, and viruses. Always dilute apple cider vinegar! It is pungent stuff. I recommend using a mixture of one part vinegar to four parts water. Apply to your face with cotton or a spritzer. No need to wash it off.

Coconut oil is an amazing body moisturizer that glides on easily and soaks in, leaving you hydrated for hours. It's antibacterial and antifungal, meaning it will help heal rashes, scars, infections, and acne. Coconut oil is full of healthy fats and antioxidants, so it offers a lot of nutrition for your skin.

Apply coconut oil right after you shower, when your pores are hydrated and ready. Scoop out a heaping tablespoon or two and spread away. For some people, coconut oil is better for the body and doesn't make their face as happy—so test it on your body first and then try applying a smaller amount to your face.

Go Virgin

When selecting oils (for your cooking and your skin), look for organic, unrefined, cold-pressed, and/or extra-virgin varieties.

Organic: The raw ingredients have not been genetically modified and were grown without (most) synthetic fertilizers and pesticides. Facilities that produce organic ingredients must also use certified organic cleaners and maintain strict sourcing records.

Unrefined: The oil has not been processed to remove impurities or to neutralize its natural scent or flavor. Synonyms include "raw," "virgin," or "pure." If you see the word *cold-pressed* on the label, that's like unrefined with bonus points.

Cold-pressed: The oil has been processed without heat that goes above 120 degrees Fahrenheit.

Extra-virgin: The oil has been both cold-pressed and processed using no chemicals.

Olive oil is a light moisturizer that's great for the face and is especially affordable. It is super-versatile and can be paired with many other ingredients effectively—as you will soon discover! Olive oil protects against sun damage and skin cancer. And it's so gentle that even the most sensitive human on the planet is probably not allergic to it. Use olive oil like coconut oil, except more freely on your face and in your hair.

Ground oats or ground almonds are gentle exfoliants that leave skin super-soft. Opt for almonds if you are gluten-free—sometimes oats have traces of gluten if they're processed in factories that also process wheat. Both of these ingredients are incredibly soothing and healing to the skin, and they reduce inflammation (the root of most skin evils). The simplest way to use oats is to pour a heaping cupful into a warm bath and soak.

Baking soda is a great spot treatment, toothpaste ingredient, deep cleanser for getting rid of shampoo buildup in hair, and odor fighter (think foot scrub!). You may have heard of the old remedy of putting toothpaste on a blemish. The baking soda in old-fashioned toothpaste was the active ingredient that made it work. The best way to use baking soda is as a once-in-a-while zit treatment. Make a paste with water and dab it on a blemish. Or spread onto a stinky area, leave on for however long you'd like (even overnight), then rinse.

Honey kills bacteria while soothing and moisturizing skin. It's also anti-inflammatory and hydrating to your pores. Honey makes a great addition to any exfoliant or mask—it even makes a great stand-alone mask. Rub it onto your face and leave on for a chunk of time (not overnight, unless you want a sticky pillowcase!), then rinse with warm water. You may need a washcloth to get it all off.

Shea butter is a very rich moisturizer. A little bit goes a long way, leaving your skin hydrated for up to a full day. Shea butter has a natural SPF of 6 and absorbs some ultraviolet radiation. All shea butter comes from Africa and most of it is fair trade, but it's a good idea to check the label. The simplest way to use shea butter is straight on your face or body, but it is really thick and can take a while to soak in, so I recommend the Super-Rich Cream recipe on page 180 to turn it into a lighter alternative.

Coarse sugar makes a great body scrub. It melts quickly in water, leaving the skin cleansed and smooth. Have you heard of those crazy, expensive glycolic acid chemical peels? That's a synthetic version of sugar. So skip that junk and scrub down with sugar when you want shiny, clear, fresh skin. The easiest way to use sugar is to scrub it on while in the shower. You can also use it on your face, but don't be too vigorous— just pat!

Aloe vera speeds up your skin's ability to heal, moisturizes it, helps it create fresh new cells, fights inflammation and itchiness, and is high in antioxidants. I'm not really sure why aloe is not treated as if it has special powers, because it really does. It's best to get it fresh from the leaf (many health food stores sell aloe leaves, and it makes a super-easy house plant); just cut it open and apply the gooey insides to your skin. You can also get it in gel or juice form in the supplement section of your local natural grocery.

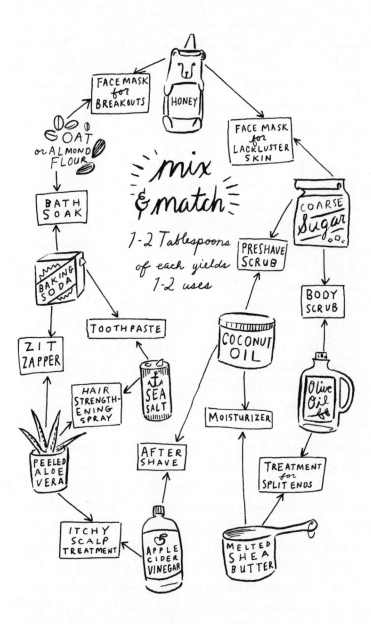

FACE MASK for BREAKOUTS

HONEY

FACE MASK for LACKLUSTER SKIN

OAT or ALMOND FLOUR

mix & match

1-2 Tablespoons of each yields 1-2 uses

COARSE Sugar

BATH SOAK

PRESHAVE SCRUB

BAKING SODA

BODY SCRUB

TOOTHPASTE

COCONUT OIL

ZIT ZAPPER

Olive Oil

HAIR STRENGTH-ENING SPRAY

SEA SALT

MOISTURIZER

PEELED ALOE VERA

AFTER SHAVE

TREATMENT for SPLIT ENDS

ITCHY SCALP TREATMENT

APPLE CIDER VINEGAR

MELTED SHEA BUTTER

GET COOKING

Now comes the part you've been waiting for: it's time to create your new skin-care regimen! What's great about making your own products is that it puts you in full control. You can keep your routine however you want it, but you'll always have the inexpensive, effective products that come right from your kitchen.

When I first started exploring the world of DIY skin care, I learned two annoying things very quickly: not all recipes are created equal, and not all recipes are as easy as they look. I became so frustrated with how often my experiments totally and utterly failed, even though they weren't that experimental at all—I was following recipes exactly as I found them. Eventually, I put it together that the recipes are not always actually tested ahead of time. Other times, a complex recipe can be incredibly temperamental. I've solved that problem here for you by testing all of the recipes thoroughly—I don't want you to go through what I did.

Additionally, there is no soap making in this book. That is super-complex stuff, and it's a little difficult to do in your kitchen. Homemade soap and emulsion-based lotions (also complex) aren't really my speed, but if you master these recipes and want to go further, I encourage you to seek out a craft class and go for it. But that's not what this book is about. This book is about simple recipes made from ingredients found in your kitchen or at your health-food store. I kept them easy and fast. I want you to actually do them, whether or not you consider yourself DIY-inclined.

It's important to know some facts about product making before you start. These rules will help you become sort of like your own apothecary. You'll eventually be able to alter recipes, explore new ingredients, and even save something that just didn't come out right. For now, here are the rules:

The bacteria that can spoil your products need *water* to live and grow. Keep this in mind with all of your concoctions. Water-based products won't last longer than a few days. So if you're mixing hydrosols (such as rosewater or distilled witch hazel) with oils or butters or fresh veggies and fruits, the products will not last very long. You can store them in the fridge for a couple of days, max. My recipes include a range of shorter and longer shelf lives.

The same is true for fresh vegetables and fruits. We're going to use fun ingredients like tomatoes and lemons and peaches, but they will spoil in the product even faster than they will on their own. Especially if water is added.

If a product goes bad, it's not dangerous, it's just yucky and may make you break out—you definitely, definitely don't want to use it if you have a cut. So just don't risk it. You'll know it's bad because it will smell rancid or spoiled, just like bad olive oil or rotting fruit.

Always dilute "strong" ingredients. When you are starting out, do this more than you think you need to. Strong ingredients include vinegars, essential oils, and lemon. Remember: a strong ingredient will have a strong smell. Dilute essential oils with a good "carrier oil," like sweet almond or (untoasted) sesame. Dilute vinegar and lemon with water.

Be aware that skin allergies are different from internal allergies. So your insides may love coconut oil, but your skin may hate it. Before using it in a recipe, test each ingredient by putting it on a small patch of skin, like the inside of your arm. Leave it for a few minutes. If your skin turns red or itchy, skip it.

When melting butters and waxes, a double boiler is not

absolutely necessary, but it does help you control heat. In a pinch, you can hold a smaller pot with your ingredients slightly submerged in a larger pot of boiling water, and stir constantly. Or throw the ingredients in a regular pot and keep the heat as low as possible, stirring a lot to keep them from scorching.

A product you whip up that is totally natural will change consistency over time. As long as you've followed the rules in the recipes, it's okay and still lovely to use.

Ingredients can be mixed and matched, so feel free to play! Remember that everything in these recipes is easy to find and affordable—and generally edible! Ideally, if you buy almond meal for a product and don't like what it does for your skin, you can look up a recipe for it and bake some cookies.

When all else fails, don't freak, just tweak. You can't really ruin any of these products. Just play with whatever comes out until you like it. If it's dry, add more liquid, if it's oily add more dry ingredients. I know it can seem scary (like cooking), but it's really much simpler. And even a product that looks like a total disaster will work wonders, unlike that burned dinner you had to throw out.

Fresher is always better for your skin, so don't you dare buy a huge cart of ingredients and then use them for only one recipe. In fact, skim through all of the recipes and try to complement skin-care recipes with food recipes you'd like to try, or with whatever ingredients you already have handy. Making a pumpkin soup or pie? Perfect, you can whip up a mask that you wear while you bake it!

In general, avoid using anything on open cuts and wounds. DIY or not, most ingredients will aggravate a wound and slow down its healing. Wash gently and regularly with natural soap and wait until it heals. Then DIY away, especially to help the scarring.

Don't get too overwhelmed about finding jars and bottles. Start with your empty beauty products. Wash the containers well and reuse them. If that doesn't work, check out the dollar store. There is a great selection of travel-size containers, which are perfect for the amount of product you'll be making. I'm also a big fan of Ball glass jars; they come in all shapes and sizes and are manufactured in the United States!

ONCE YOU'VE GOT A handle on the basics and have started to see your skin glow from your new products, you can feel free to play with what's in your kitchen cabinets and grocery store aisles, all on your own.

There are different versions of cleansers, toners, exfoliants, and more. I even got a few friends, creators of their own amazing natural skin-care lines, to pitch in. You may recognize their brands. All of these recipes are great to try during your skin cleanse. They are also safe and gentle enough to add to your daily regimen and effective enough to replace some of your current products. Find your favorites and use them as often as you would like!

All right, all right, let's get started already!

FACE

Ah, the face. You know when you go to the gym and a disproportionate number of people are doing bicep curls? That's because it's so easy for us to see our biceps. They are known as superficial muscles, or "show muscles." As one of my personal trainer friends used to say, "If you want to get girls, do your curls!"

The face is the bicep of our skin because we put so much work into making it look good. But generally, we should be much gentler with facial skin than body skin, so the recipes for your face will be calming, healing, and subtle—yet effective. I promise, you'll be shocked by how happy your skin will be!

Cleansers

Cleansing is an essential step in your daily routine. Sure, you can wash with water and get great skin. But sometimes a cleanser is needed to get rid of dirt and oil. It's especially important to use a cleanser if you live in a polluted environment or sweat a lot. If you have extremely sensitive skin, you should cleanse slightly less often, perhaps once a day rather than twice. If you are dealing with acne and blemishes even after taking a break from your products, you should cleanse more often, but still not more than twice a day. And of course, these recipes work for all skin types.

CLEANSING MUD

This "mud" is great for people with skin that is prone to acne, redness, or painful chapping. Coconut milk is incredibly soothing, and cinnamon is a "strong" ingredient; but when diluted, cinnamon kills bacteria and fights acne. And clay—in the beauty aisle at natural grocery stores and drugstores—is detoxifying and purifying; it will pull dirt from your skin, which then gets rinsed away!

¼ teaspoon powdered cinnamon
1 tablespoon dry clay
3 tablespoons coconut milk

Mix cinnamon and clay in a small bowl. Pour in coconut milk, stirring the liquid into the dry powder evenly (use a fork or whisk to break up any clumps). Eventually, it will become a paste. Apply like a wet face scrub with a cotton ball or with your hands. You can leave it on until it dries or rinse off immediately. The mud dries out quickly, so this recipe makes only about two applications. You'll want to make a fresh batch each time you use it.

CLARIFYING ROSEWATER CLEANSER

This rosewater cleanser is a real miracle worker, and it's perfect for washing up after a sweaty workout, for treating skin in the middle of a breakout, and for those times when your skin feels as if it could use some softening. Rosewater offers many benefits in one—it's soothing, moisturizing, and toning. Lemon juice is conditioning and helps smooth out uneven skin tone. Carrot-seed oil provides a super-deep cleanse and also moisturizes your skin (you can usually find carrot-seed oil in the beauty aisle at a health-food store, and it's also easy to find online). This rinse will sting a little while you're using it and for a few minutes after, but don't fret! That's how you know it's working.

¼ cup rosewater
¼ cup fresh lemon juice (about one full lemon)
5 to 10 drops carrot-seed oil

Pour rosewater and lemon juice into a small jar (that comes with a lid) and add the carrot-seed oil. Put the lid on the jar and shake it well. Apply to face with cotton. You can leave it on or rinse it off. Store in the sealed jar in a cool dark place or in your fridge—the carrot-seed oil will preserve this wash for many weeks, and the recipe will yield over two dozen uses, but try to use it within a month!

A Rose by Any Other Name

Beware: some "rosewater" is just water with added rose fragrance. Check the label—the best (and most expensive) rosewater is made from distilled rose petals. Other rosewater is basically essential oil mixed with water—it's not as good as distilled, but it's easy to find and it's still pretty great.

Calming Aloe Cleanser

This cleanser is perfect for people with extremely sensitive skin that breaks out from everything. Mânuka honey is produced by honeybees that have eaten tea tree pollen (tea tree is a powerful antiseptic), so this honey is loaded with antibacterial properties. Aloe is a gentle moisturizer that helps calm the skin and fight inflammation, and the addition of lavender oil makes this cleanser as calming for the mind as it is for the body. Try to use fresh aloe, but you can also buy pure aloe juice or aloe gel—meaning, made from only aloe and nothing else.

1 tablespoon fresh aloe from the leaf or aloe juice
½ tablespoon mânuka honey
2 to 3 drops lavender essential oil

If you are using fresh aloe, cut through the skin of the leaf, exposing the inside so you can easily access all of it. Scoop with a knife or spoon, the way you would an avocado. Place the aloe, honey, and lavender oil in a small bowl and stir well (or, if you're using fresh aloe, whisk together with a fork) so that the honey melts into the aloe and lavender. Apply with clean hands or cotton. Rinse well (it will be sticky!). Store extra cleanser in a jar with a lid; it will last a few months. It makes enough for about six to eight uses.

BALANCING OIL CLEANSER

Despite what you may believe about applying oil to your face, oil cleansing is actually great for all skin types. If you have oily skin, your insides and outsides probably aren't hydrated enough—your body tries to make up for what it's lacking by producing extra oil. I don't love castor oil, which is a popular ingredient in many oil cleansers, because it can be very harsh. Hazelnut oil is gentler, moisturizing, and offers astringent properties, helping to regulate sebum production. Avocado oil is a deep moisturizer and contains sterolins—natural steroids that boost collagen and treat age spots. And sesame oil is a light oil that also kills bad bacteria on your skin, leaving you nice and clean.

1 tablespoon hazelnut oil
1 tablespoon avocado oil
1 tablespoon sesame oil

Pour oils into a small bottle, screw on the lid, and shake. Massage the oil onto your face with your hands and then rinse away with warm water or your regular face wash. You can also leave the oil on (I wouldn't recommend doing this if you're going to wear makeup, but you can do it before bed)—just gently pat with a towel to remove the excess. This recipe makes a little over one ounce (about a dozen uses), but it'll last up to six months, so feel free to double it.

SQUEAKY-CLEAN FOAMING FACE WASH

All right, I know you want a nice sudsy cleanser, so I'm giving in. We're going to use castile soap and make the gentlest of gentle foaming face washes. Unless you are getting sweaty a lot or live in a very polluted environment, you don't *need* to use a sudsy face wash regularly. But for those of you living in a big city or addicted to hot yoga class, I get it. The jojoba oil in this recipe will make the soap even gentler and more moisturizing, and will also fight inflammation. Tea tree oil is a terrific bug killer; it fights infections and fungus and reduces inflammation almost instantly. Use this face wash on days when you wore a lot of makeup, worked in a coal mine, slathered on sunscreen, or took that yoga class.

½ cup of unscented castile soap (I love Dr. Bronner's, who doesn't?)
2 tablespoons jojoba oil
10 drops tea tree oil

Pour your soap and oil into a bottle with a lid or pump, then add tea tree oil. Seal and shake well—it'll get bubbly, but also beautifully creamy and luxurious. Let it sit overnight before using, and shake before each use. Apply as you would your regular face cleanser—it will make a thin, sudsy soap. Will last a few months; just make sure to keep water out.

BREAKOUT-BUSTING SODA PASTE

This paste is great for acne-prone and oily skin. Baking soda will kill the bacteria on your face that's causing breakouts, and sweet almond oil will stop the baking soda from drying you out. Sweet almond oil will also kill the bacteria in your oily pores. It's extremely gentle, and it'll soak in and hydrate your skin. This paste also makes a great spot treatment and will zap a zit in no time.

1 tablespoon baking soda
Slightly less than 1 tablespoon sweet almond oil

Combine both ingredients in a small jar or bowl and stir well to make an oily paste. Gently scrub onto face in small, circular motions and rinse clean. Or apply to blemishes and leave on overnight to reduce redness and inflammation. Rinse off in the morning before washing your face like usual. This recipe will make over a dozen uses, and it can be stored for a few months.

Toners

Toner and astringent are not an essential part of your routine, but they can be an amazing addition. Technically a toner helps with dry skin and astringent helps with oily skin, but no need to overthink it. What good (in other words, *natural*) versions of both do is balance your skin. They correct your pH and protect your acid mantle. They kill bacteria and soothe red, splotchy skin. You should use less toner and astringent as you get older, and you should also skip them if you are extremely sensitive, as they will cause an increase in blood flow to your skin. If you do not struggle with breakouts or an uneven skin tone, then these recipes are not essential for you, they are treats to use once in a while for a little pick-me-up!

CLOCK-STOPPING ELECTROLYTE TONER

This is a great toner for people with aging skin. Peaches are high in vitamin C, which boosts the production of collagen in your skin, making it appear more youthful. Coconut water contains cytokinins, plant hormones that keep your skin smooth and elastic. They may even fight wrinkles. Coconut water is also a great hydrator for your outsides just like it is for your insides!

1 small, very ripe, de-pitted peach, mashed
½ cup coconut water

Combine peach with coconut water in a medium-size jar, seal, and shake well (if you wanted to make the texture smoother, you could also use a blender). Apply with cotton and rinse clean. Keep it sealed in your fridge for up to a few days. It will make about two dozen uses.

Tightening Bloody Mary Toner

Tomatoes are full of antioxidants and are also very acidic. Acid in your body isn't always the greatest, but when it comes to your skin, acid is a very good thing. Tomatoes dry up the excess oil that's already there and fight acne by preventing your skin from producing too much oil. You can even take a slice of tomato and coat your skin with the juice—it'll work as a toner all on its own. Vodka actually makes for a great toner—it cleanses and tightens the skin (although I'm not a fan of alcohol as an ingredient in commercial products). And yes, you can sip on this, too.

3 tablespoons tomato juice (fresh is best, but jarred or canned is okay, too)
1 teaspoon apple cider vinegar
1 teaspoon vodka

Combine all ingredients into a small jar with a lid, seal, and shake well. Apply with cotton and rinse. Keep it sealed in your fridge for up to a few days. It will yield about a dozen uses.

DIY Tomato Juice:
It's super-simple to make your own tomato juice—just roughly chop a ripe tomato and transfer it (seeds and juice included) to a blender and blend until smooth. Or throw the chopped tomato into a bowl and mash it with a potato masher or a fork. Strain through a thin-meshed sieve and voilà! You have the base for a brunch cocktail *or* an astringent.

BRIGHTENING ASTRINGENT

This is a great astringent for itchy, irritated, or acne-prone skin. Witch hazel reduces swelling, fights bacteria, and helps to heal wounds. It also tightens the skin and helps rid the skin of excess oil. Chamomile tea helps even out dark patches, soothes irritation, and reduces inflammation. It also helps heal wounds and prevent scarring.

1 tablespoon witch hazel
1 tablespoon brewed and cooled strong chamomile tea
(I like to do two bags in one cup of water,
letting it steep for fifteen to twenty minutes.)

Pour the witch hazel and chamomile tea into a small regular bottle or a small spritzer bottle, and apply either with cotton or by spritzer. This astringent can be left on if your skin is happy with it (it's incredibly gentle), or rinsed off. The recipe will make enough for about five applications, but it will last only a couple of days—so store it in the fridge and use it a few times a day until you run out.

MAKEUP REMOVER

You already know how important it is to take off your makeup! Of course, you can use simple kitchen-cabinet oils to remove your makeup, but oils feel heavy to some people (even the light ones), and if they get in your eyes while you're removing eye makeup, things can get a little blurry. The aloe in this remover cuts the oil. Sweet almond oil is gentle and will kill bacteria as it's wiping away your makeup, so you don't need to wash it off.

2 tablespoons sweet almond oil
1 tablespoon aloe vera leaf, juice, or gel

Combine ingredients in a small jar with a lid, seal, and shake well. Apply to your face with cotton and leave on. The remover will settle and separate, so shake well every time you use it. You will get about a dozen applications from this recipe, depending on how much makeup you're removing. Store in a cool dark place and use within two to three weeks. Feel free to use it as a moisturizer also!

Moisturizers

The most crucial step of all, in my humble opinion, moisturizing is something that all of us should be doing, no matter our skin type or age. Moisturizing becomes significantly more important as you age, but you can greatly impact the future health of your skin by starting early. Many of us have skin that is parched for moisture because commercial lotions are full of chemicals that are very drying, and because many lotions contain a lot of water. Water leaves your skin drier when it evaporates (that's why washing with just water can sometimes make you feel a little tight), so it should appear as an ingredient only in your other products, and not in your moisturizer. Oils hydrate your skin—they do not clog your pores.

I've given you only two moisturizers here. That's because they really work, for all skin types, and there is no need to make hydration complicated. They can both be used on the face or body, and they can be rotated in with your own moisturizer or a simple one-ingredient routine like coconut oil or olive oil.

SUPER-RICH CREAM

I believe that shea butter is the single greatest skin-care ingredient. It changed my life, and it is essentially the reason I started S.W. Basics. Shea butter is incredibly healing, and it improves virtually every skin ailment. With mine, those improvements happened overnight. I love cocoa butter because it smells like (and is!) chocolate. It is also very moisturizing and gentle. The addition of avocado oil makes this cream just a touch less rich, so it's easier to spread around and soak in. The result is a super-luxurious staple that is also a powerful moisturizer and skin treatment.

¼ cup shea butter

¼ cup cocoa butter

2 tablespoons avocado oil

Melt shea butter and cocoa butter in a small pot on the stovetop (ideally in a double boiler) until completely liquefied, stirring well. Remove from heat and stir in avocado oil. Allow to completely cool, and then cover and place in the fridge until it solidifies, usually one to two hours. After an hour, give it a stir—the texture should be like butter. Transfer to a lidded jar and use within six to eight months, because your hands will introduce bacteria into the product that will make it spoil. Heads up: this recipe will make your pot very oily; you may need to soak it in some hot, soapy water to clean. Also, it will make enough uses to last you that entire six to eight months.

LIGHT MOISTURIZING FACE AND BODY OIL

Grapeseed oil is light and soaks into the skin very easily. It's also slightly astringent, so it acts as a toner as well. You can find it in the cooking aisle at the grocery store. Pumpkin-seed oil is not only hydrating, it is also full of vitamins and minerals. It reduces fine lines and stops moisture from leaving your skin. Flaxseed oil is amazing for eczema and psoriasis because it is a strong anti-inflammatory. It also has the highest ratio of omega-3s to omega-6s of any oil, so it will strengthen your skin and make it look younger.

½ cup grapeseed oil
¼ cup pumpkin-seed oil
1 tablespoon flaxseed oil

Pour the oils into a regular bottle or pump bottle and shake well. Pour or pump out a little and apply with your hands. Keep this sealed in the fridge for up to one month—just remember to warm it up in your hands before you apply! The recipe will make enough for you to coat your body with it three times a day for the whole month.

How to Moisturize

The right time to moisturize is anytime as far as I'm concerned, but it's best to use oils on the face and body right after toweling off from the shower, so the water already on your skin goes into your pores and stays there. I also prefer fully liquid moisturizers for my body because they spread more easily and quickly. I think solid cream is great for the face (especially around the eye area and on any dry patches); solid cream is good for dry areas on the body, too. But moisturize in whichever way makes you happy, and don't forget your hair might love some of these hydrating ingredients, too!

Exfoliants and Masks

And now to the face treats! These are the recipes for when you want to give your skin some extra glow, when you're staying in on a Friday night, or when you forgot to make a present for the baby shower that's . . . tomorrow.

The main difference between an exfoliant and a mask is how they do their work. With an exfoliant, you scrub it on and activate it as you use it; with a mask, you apply it to your skin and give it some time to work its magic. Both will technically exfoliate your skin—meaning they pull out toxins, dirt, and oil, slough off dead skin cells, and get your blood flowing. Beware that sometimes masks and exfoliants will cause you to break out, especially if it's been a while and there's a lot of dirt coming out of your pores. Don't fret, because a good recipe will also accelerate the healing of said breakouts. And obviously all of these recipes are brilliant.

Feel free to experiment with your exfoliation: you can scrub first, rinse clean, then apply the same mixture and leave it on for a little while as a mask. Or vice versa—apply a mask and then scrub it in before removing (this is my favorite way to exfoliate). Remember your skin may need some time to get used to exfoliating, so be gentle. I like to follow my masks immediately with moisturizer. At the very least, massage some olive oil into your skin to fill your bare pores with healthy and nourishing hydration.

As a bonus, all of these masks and exfoliants can also be used on the rest of your body. So make extra for the shower!

DETOX MASK

Chickpeas are an amazing detoxifier. They pull out harmful toxins, neutralize free radicals, heal sun damage, and generally energize your skin (and your insides, too, of course). For this recipe, you can mash cooked chickpeas or canned chickpeas, or you can hydrate chickpea flour (often called garbanzo flour). All three will work about the same, just use your judgment with how much water to add. Turmeric regulates oil production, reduces inflammation, and heals scars, especially those from acne. This mask can be a little drying, so definitely follow with a moisturizer.

1 tablespoon chickpea flour or mashed chickpeas
Generous pinch of turmeric powder (enough to tint the
   mixture yellowish)
1 tablespoon water

Combine chickpeas and turmeric in a small bowl, then stir in the water. If you're using cooked or canned chickpeas, make sure to really mix in the turmeric. You can apply with your fingers—it will feel as if you are putting hummus on your face (you kind of are). For maximum detox benefit, let it dry before washing it off. Keep it sealed in your fridge for up to a week. Will make two to three applications.

Skin Feast Mask

Brown rice flour is a great (gluten-free!) mask ingredient. It is full of nutrients, and it soaks up excess oil. Avocado helps to balance your oil production by "feeding" your skin a healthy fat. Apple juice also combats oily skin. This mask is incredibly gentle and rich; there will be no sting, only soothe.

1 tablespoon brown rice flour
½ an avocado
1 tablespoon apple juice (fresh pressed, if possible)

In a small bowl, mash avocado with a fork and sprinkle in rice flour, stirring until you've created a paste. Add apple juice and stir well. Apply mask and allow to dry for best results. Rinse with warm water. This recipe will make two or three applications but will spoil, so store in fridge and use it quickly.

Dessert Mask

Cocoa powder (or cacao, for you fancy folks) helps repair and prevent cell damage because it is full of antioxidants. Sea salt kills bacteria and is great for blemishes. The olive oil will make the salt and cocoa gentler on your skin, while also leaving you moisturized after the exfoliation.

4 teaspoons cocoa powder
½ teaspoon sea salt
2 teaspoons olive oil

Mix cocoa powder and salt in a small bowl, then stir in olive oil to create a paste. Apply with your fingers and leave on for as long as you'd like. The sea salt may start to sting over time as it works its magic. Rinse carefully—this mask will stain a washcloth. Makes one to two uses and can sit out on your counter for a few days.

Deep Sea Hydrating "Strips"

This one's for all you dry-skinned ladies out there. Seaweed is so good for you internally and externally—it draws toxins from the skin, is full of B vitamins, clears away dead skin cells, and leaves you hydrated and dewy-fresh. Cucumbers are high in antioxidants and in vitamins C and K, which means they combat inflammation and aging. Cukes also have lots of vitamin A (natural retinol), which will even your skin tone and help you glow. Coffee is full of antioxidants and healthy oil for your skin. You're going to be using a little bit of brewed coffee for this recipe, since I know you have some every day (you junkie). This recipe is slightly advanced but still really fun.

½ cup cooled coffee
½ peeled cucumber, roughly chopped
1 sheet kombu seaweed

Add the coffee and cucumber to a blender and blend until smooth. Pour mixture into a shallow bowl and add the sheet of seaweed. Soak until it is completely rehydrated. To apply, first put cotton into the cuke and coffee mixture and dab it on your skin. Then tear the kombu into strips and firmly press them all over your face, focusing on the under-eye area, forehead, nose, and any dry patches. Leave on and hang out, making sure to scare as many people as possible while you look like an underwater monster. When finished, peel off and discard strips of kombu and rinse clean. When you see how amazing your skin looks, feel free to toss the gross drugstore "pore strips" from your cabinet. Makes one use.

Oil-Balancing Mayo Mask

I almost skipped using mayo as a mask ingredient for two reasons. The first is that it stinks and the idea of putting it on your skin grosses some people out. The second is that on its own, mayo already contains a lot of ingredients. But then I remembered I taught you to make your own mayonnaise, and this recipe was born. The orange juice will mask the scent of the mayo wonderfully, and it also brightens the skin with its vitamin C. Corn flour is a soft exfoliant and does an amazing job of soaking up excess oil from the skin. This is a great mask to use if you're really oily.

1 tablespoon homemade mayo (or organic if you want to use store bought)
1 tablespoon orange juice (fresh is best; bottled is fine)
2 tablespoons corn flour

In a small bowl, stir together all three ingredients slowly, making sure to fully incorporate the corn flour into the wet ingredients. For best results, apply with your fingers and let dry. The corn will not melt in the solution and will be a bit grainy, so be very gentle when applying. This recipe will make about three applications, but it will spoil quickly, so store it in a sealed container in the fridge and use within a few days.

Reparative Oat-Berry Cookie Exfoliant

Mmm, now let's make the cookie of face exfoliants. This recipe is great for all skin types because it is very gentle yet just abrasive enough to provide a deep clean. You will seriously want to eat this one as you're applying it (go ahead, I won't tell). You know by now that olive oil and oats offer all kinds of benefits for your skin, and jojoba oil gently combats dryness and kills bacteria. Berries are full of potent antioxidants and collagen-boosting and skin-repairing vitamin C. Coconut flour (available at most health-food stores or gluten-free sections of grocery stores) is made from dried coconut meat that is ground into a soft powder. It soothes and smooths the skin.

3 strawberries
10 raspberries
1 teaspoon ground oats, aka oat flour
¼ cup coconut flour
2 tablespoons olive oil or jojoba oil

Using a small bowl and the back of a fork, or a mortar and pestle, mash strawberries and raspberries together. Using a separate bowl, combine oats and coconut flour. Stir olive oil into flours, then add the mashed berries. This recipe makes a good amount, but it will spoil quickly, so try to use it all at once with your friends, partner, or kids. You will smell delicious. If you do have any leftovers, store in the fridge but toss if not used after a couple of days.

Pumpkin Pie Glow Mask

(courtesy of Jordan Pacitti, see box below)

This mask is great for removing dead skin and unclogging pores. The flaxseeds provide a gentle physical exfoliation while the pumpkin enzymes and lactose in the yogurt offer a chemical exfoliation. Add in raw honey for super-charged hydration, and you'll be good to glow!

¼ cup full-fat Greek yogurt
1 tablespoon raw honey
¼ cup pumpkin purée (not pumpkin pie mix)
1 tablespoon ground flaxseeds or flax meal

In a small bowl, stir together yogurt and honey. Once the honey is fully incorporated, add in pumpkin purée and then stir in the flaxseeds. Use your fingers to apply and leave on until you feel it drying, then rinse with warm water. Makes a few uses; store extra in the fridge for up to a week.

Yelp a Facialist

I have a confession—I've never gotten a facial in my entire life! With my sensitive skin, I've always found them terrifying. That's why I created recipes to give you the experience of a facial at home. But people ask me all the time about the "real" thing, so I asked my friend and sought-after facialist **Jordan Pacitti** for the inside scoop. He is an amazing natural facialist based in Seattle, Washington, with a cult following. He made the switch to natural after seeing client after client with what he calls "schizophrenic skin"—skin that seemed really oily on the surface but was actually dry and damaged. All of those clients had been getting harsh facials regularly, so he decided to create a natural alternative. Here's his advice:

Facial treatments have seen an increase in "result-oriented" therapies over the past thirty years, ranging from microdermabrasion and alpha hydroxy acids to lasers, lights, and microcurrents. Even with all of these new treatments and products, skin conditions such as acne, rosacea, and pigmentation are on the rise. The truth is that we are simply doing too much to our skin—breaking it down and thinning it by overscrubbing (with plastic beads, no less), overpeeling and overinjecting. It's important to build the skin up and stop breaking it down. Here are my DO's and DON'T's for facials:

For the best results, DO continue going to an aesthetician you already like. That way the two of you can develop a long-term plan.

DON'T go for monthly chemical peels. While acids remove the top layer of skin and give you an immediate glow, they can also thin the skin over time. This is because they weaken the skin, creating a mix of dehydration, excessive oiliness, severe redness, and irritation.

DO look for facials that use LED light therapy. This is one modern-day treatment that I highly recommend.

It will regenerate skin tissue, stimulate the production of collagen and elastin, kill acne bacteria, even skin tone, and reduce redness. There isn't much that this magic light can't do. Oh yeah . . . it releases serotonin, the happiness chemical, in the brain, too!

DON'T let the smell of essential oils fool you. Make sure you choose a spa, private practice, or clinic that uses *truly* natural and botanical skin care. This requires you to do a little research. Find out what line they will be using and research the ingredients.

DO get a deep cleanse. A major component of any facial is extractions. Make sure your aesthetician is skilled in the removal of blackheads and clogged pores. While you do want extractions, make sure they are not too harsh. You may leave red and splotchy if extractions are performed incorrectly.

DON'T get a facial that uses too much electricity around your head. I feel too much agitation via electricity results in agitated skin—red, congested, bumpy, irritated. Sound familiar? Stay away from the electricity.

DO get facials that give lots of massage. Not only will massage relax the nervous system, resulting in better skin, it will also help tone, lift, and oxygenate the skin tissue. You will leave your facial feeling *and* looking amazing.

DON'T get oversold on products. When receiving a facial, ask lots of questions. If they start recommending a ton of products, ask why they would be good for you. A good aesthetician will recommend things that you need to get the results you want. They won't put you on a whole new program just to make a few bucks. If the product sounds too good to be true, it probably is. And always remember, with skin, less is more!

BODY CARE

The skin on the rest of our bodies often suffers the same ailments as our face, but it gets way less attention. The nice thing about taking care of the skin on your body is that it's slightly less sensitive than your face. You can scrub and exfoliate more vigorously; you can soak in the tub; and you can coat your body skin in luxurious oils. As with the face recipes, these body-care recipes cross over, which means you can use them everywhere and you can use them all the time.

Combination Face and Body Exfoliant

Think of this exfoliant as an at-home chemical peel minus the chemicals. (When did chemical peels become a normal thing, and why is no one talking about how crazy it is to chemically peel the skin off your face? But I digress . . .) Sugar is a great all-over exfoliant, and the vitamin C in lime makes your skin firmer and more youthful. And as you may remember, papaya is a superfood for your skin—it's high in vitamin A, will remove dead skin cells, and brightens the skin.

¼ cup papaya chunks
¼ cup coarse sugar
Juice from ½ lime

It's easiest to whip this recipe up in a blender, if you can. If not, mash the papaya with a fork in a small bowl, then mix in the sugar and the lime juice. Mix it all together to form a paste. If applying to the face, do so gently—no harsh scrubbing! Just lightly use your fingers in circular motions (stimulates blood flow). Leave on for a few minutes or for up to a half hour, then rinse clean. For your body, you can definitely scrub more vigorously. You can do this whole process in the shower (and you should, the mixture is very slippery!), but keep an eye on your drain, as it may clog. This recipe makes one use for your entire body, and it will keep for a few days in the fridge. Use the rest of your papaya, lime, and sugar as the base of a cocktail smoothie.

BODY MASK

This treatment is especially great if you have body breakouts. Both the clay and green tea will help extract dirt while feeding your skin with nutrients and antioxidants. Dry clay just means any type of clay powder made from . . . the earth. It is inexpensive and easy to find. You can use bentonite clay or French green clay, which are both popular varieties. They're all awesome.

Contents from 4 opened green tea bags
¼ cup dry clay
¼ cup warm water

Dump contents of your green tea bags into a deep bowl with the clay and stir well. Mix in warm water until it becomes a smooth, thick paste. In the shower, cover your whole body with the mixture and hang out for a minute or so before rinsing clean. This will make your bathtub look super-dirty but these ingredients will rinse away easily. This mask dries out easily, so keep it in the shower and use one or two times before tossing any excess.

Soothing Bath Soak

Sea salt is great for clearing up body breakouts—it removes dead skin cells, increases blood circulation, and kills bad bacteria on your body. The oats do the same and will also soothe sensitive or irritated skin, as will the rosemary and basil. Feel free to swap out any of the herbs with others you prefer; they're all great!

½ cup sea salt
½ cup ground oats
1 bunch fresh rosemary or fresh, washed basil
Rubber band for herbs (optional)

Mix together sea salt and oats in a large bowl and add to a hot bath, along with the herbs. Feel free to tie herbs together with a rubber band, but make sure to agitate the water so that everything brews like a big cup of tea. If you chop or tear the herbs, they will release more beneficial enzymes. You might want to cover the drainer with a thin towel or cheesecloth if you have sensitive plumbing and don't want anything to get washed down the drain. Discard herbs when you're done relaxing. Follow by showering or toweling clean and applying moisturizer, and you may need to rinse your tub out, as the salt and oats will settle.

FOOT SOAK

You may have heard how great Epsom salt is for bath time. It helps soothe sore muscles and promotes relaxation—which also makes it perfect for your overtired, overworked feet! Epsom salt is usually sold in big bags at the pharmacy, so use some for this recipe and some for a bath after a tough workout. Use fresh mint for the strongest effect, but mint tea bags work, too.

1 bunch fresh mint (or 6 mint tea bags)
About 4 quarts water
1 cup Epsom salt
30 drops peppermint oil
30 drops lavender oil
½ to 1 cup aloe juice (optional)

Squeeze mint in your hands until the leaves are bruised, add them (or your 6 tea bags) to your largest pot full of water and bring to a boil on the stove. The longer you boil, the more potent the "tea" will become, so let it go as long as you'd like. Turn off the heat, add Epsom salt, and stir until dissolved. Let this cool enough for you to handle it comfortably before adding essential oils, or they will evaporate. But don't wait too long, or it won't feel as nice on your feet. Optionally, and especially if you are feeling impatient, add ½ to 1 cup aloe juice for a soothing effect that also cools the temperature enough to get your feet in it. Pour into a basin and sink your feet in. This recipe will make one use.

Essential Oils

Ah, essential oils. No ingredient is more overvalued by hippies or undervalued by everyone else. Essential oils are like plant medicine. Think of orange oil as an orange on crack and of peppermint oil as mint times one thousand. All essential oils are extremely strong ingredients, and you should always dilute them by mixing them with something else. If you are just starting out, use only two to four drops in a recipe. If you are a pro, and you already know what your skin likes, you can probably handle a lot of them straight, but you should still dilute. Doing so is safer and will make them last longer. You can also diffuse oils to make your home smell delicious. For now, you're just going to put them in your skin-care products. You can find essential oils at your local health-food store or herb/spice/tea shops. Here are my favorites, and the ones I consider the safest for use in skin care:

Peppermint	Cardamom
Lavender	Lemongrass
Sweet orange	Patchouli
Geranium	Bergamot
Clary sage	Carrot seed
Sandalwood	Frankincense
Tea tree	

Deodorant

Rachel Winard is the owner and founder of Soapwalla, another Brooklyn-based skin-care brand that I love. She is an expert at making deodorant and has created the most famous completely natural deodorant on the market. Here, she shares two deodorant recipes with us!

DEODORANT SPRITZER

3 tablespoons pure witch hazel
2 tablespoons aloe vera gel
Large pinch baking soda (no more than ¼ teaspoon)
8 drops of your favorite deodorizing essential oil (lavender, tea tree, cedar, lemon, clary sage, lemongrass)

Add all ingredients to a small spray bottle and shake for a solid minute until the baking soda has dissolved and the essential oil is well mixed. Let stand overnight, then in the morning give it another good shake, spritz, and enjoy the rest of your day knowing you smell fresh and clean, like a flower. This recipe will last a couple of months; shake well each time you use it.

DEODORANT CREAM

3 tablespoons coconut oil
2 tablespoons corn flour, arrowroot, or tapioca starch (whatever you have lying around)
2 tablespoons baking soda
8 to 10 drops favorite deodorizing essential oil (lavender, tea tree, cedar, lemon, clary sage, lemongrass)—start small and increase as needed

Gently melt coconut oil in a small pot. Whisk in powders. Add essential oil, a few drops at a time, until you reach your desired scent and intensity. Once thoroughly mixed, place in your jar of choice, pop in the fridge for fifteen minutes until set, then schmear and be clear. This recipe will last a couple of months, but it may separate. Just stir well before using if it does!

PERFUME

Most sprayed perfumes quickly evaporate off your skin—and if your fragrance does stick around, it's probably got lots of chemicals in it to make that happen. Solid perfume is the way to go because you won't need any preservatives to hold the fragrance to your skin. Beeswax is great because it's incredibly gentle and it sits on top of the skin for a long period of time. You can find it at many health food stores, craft stores, and at the honey stand at your local farmers' market.

1 tablespoon organic beeswax pellets
1 tablespoon jojoba oil
30 to 40 drops patchouli oil, of course (just kidding!)—so
    many options, choose from the essential oil chart and feel
    free to mix

This recipe will make you feel like a chemist. In a small pot, melt down the beeswax and add the jojoba oil. Pour out the mixture into a container with a lid (like an empty lip balm tin), then add essential oils. The wax needs to be in the cooling stages before you add the essential oil or it will cook off completely. Watch carefully: once you pour the mixture into a container, it will solidify faster than you can imagine! Apply with your fingers where you would put on perfume. Will last up to a year and make lots and lots and lots of uses.

TOOTHPASTE

It seems like the verdict is still out on the safety of fluoride, so I like to rotate this DIY toothpaste into my regimen. Sometimes I'll use it every other day; sometimes I'll go natural for a week straight. Baking soda is an abrasive, but a very mild and gentle one. Have you heard of oil pulling? It's all the rage these days—and coconut oil is often used. It kills bacteria in your mouth and creates a soapy effect that leaves teeth squeaky clean. Add essential oils for a nice scent, plus a little more antibacterial action.

1 tablespoon melted coconut oil
2 tablespoons baking soda
5 to 10 drops: peppermint oil, spearmint oil, clove oil,
*   or cinnamon oil*

In a small bowl, mix coconut oil and baking soda well, then add drops of essential oil and stir. Use like your normal toothpaste. If you make sure not to dip your toothbrush directly into the paste (scoop it out with a clean utensil instead), this recipe will last for a few months, though it may separate and require some stirring. It can be stored in a small open or sealed jar in your bathroom, and will make about a month's worth for brushing twice a day.

Mouthwash

Did you know that using a chemical mouthwash was recently linked to an unhealthy spike in blood pressure?[25] It's true. The synthetic ingredients are so insanely strong that they kill everything in your mouth, even healthy bacteria that help contribute to healthy blood pressure. So my recommendation is that you skip the hard-core stuff, and instead use this natural version only once in a while. Aloe juice and baking soda both fight plaque and gingivitis. Baking soda also whitens teeth. The peppermint will leave you with a super-clean, minty mouth.

¼ cup aloe juice
¼ cup water
1½ teaspoons baking soda
2 to 8 drops peppermint oil

Mix all ingredients in a bottle or cup and shake or stir well. Be careful with the peppermint oil—add a drop or two at a time and smell to decide how potent you would like this to be. (If you're curious about oil pulling, this is a good recipe to add as much coconut oil or sesame oil to as you would like.) Use like regular mouthwash. Shake well each time you use this product, and although it'll make enough uses for about two weeks, it will keep for about a month. Can be stored in your bathroom cabinet.

LIP BALM

Ladies and gentlemen, this is the exact recipe for our original S.W. Basics lip balm. How's that for transparency? When I first discovered it was this easy to make lip balm, I laughed out loud. Or maybe I didn't, but that's how it felt. Go look at how many ingredients are in your lip balm(s). Way more than you need. You need only these three ingredients to make a creamy, healing balm. And it'll last forever.

1 tablespoon beeswax pellets
1 tablespoon cocoa butter
1 tablespoon coconut oil
Several drops of essential oil of choice (optional)

Melt all three ingredients in a double boiler over low heat. Pour mixture into a little container that has a lid (like the old tin that a store-bought lip balm came in). Remember that if you want to add scent, you should put the essential oils in at the very end. Also, be ready when you turn the heat off—the mixture will cool and harden almost instantly. You'll want to be ready to pour the second it's melted. This lip balm will last about a year and will have a million uses.

LIP SCRUB

While it's true that a really gorgeous lip balm like that one you just made will heal dry lips, sometimes you just can't manage the chap. You live somewhere that is so brutal on your skin and lips that the lip balm can't keep up, or you're experiencing the coldest winter of your life. Leave it to an amazing lip scrub to help. It'll remove the dead skin that is chapped and moisturize your rosy lips underneath.

1 tablespoon honey
1 tablespoon brown sugar
1 teaspoon coconut oil

    In a small bowl, mix the honey and brown sugar, then add the coconut oil and stir. Press and scrub onto lips. Don't worry if it gets in your mouth because it'll taste delicious. Rinse clean, scrubbing while you rinse. Your lips will be a little sensitive after you scrub, so make sure to apply that lip balm you made, or an equally high-quality one. Makes about four uses. Will store for a few weeks but will harden over time.

HAIR

HAIR MASK/SHAMPOO

People have been asking for S.W. Basics to make a shampoo since the day we launched. If I could make this recipe last on a shelf, it is the exact shampoo that I would sell. That's how amazing it is. The shampoo you use now, natural or not, is made up of harsh detergents that are brutal on your hair and even more brutal on your scalp. But non-shampoo soap isn't the right pH for your hair, either, so it can be drying. It's quite the conundrum! Enter the best DIY product of your whole life. Coconut milk is incredibly moisturizing, so it'll combat the castile soap in the recipe, which is needed to actually clean your hair. The clay will help clear extra dirt from your hair and detox your scalp. You're going to be amazed by this recipe, I promise.

⅓ cup castile soap
¼ cup coconut milk
4 tablespoons dry clay

In a small bowl, mix together all three ingredients, stirring gently to stop mixture from foaming. Use instead of your normal shampoo up to twice a week. You can also wash your face with this mixture while you're shampooing. It will dry out and spoil quickly, so try to use it all during one shower.

HAIR CONDITIONER

This is another recipe I would love to bottle up and sell. DIY conditioners are usually full of oil, but I think it's very difficult to get oil out of your hair. I prefer this recipe, which is still very conditioning but really light and easy to rinse out. Beer is full of B vitamins, repairs damaged hair, and adds volume. The fatty acid content of eggs helps moisturize and condition your hair, and apple cider vinegar will help make your hair shiny and also clear you of scalp issues and buildup. The nice thing about this conditioner is that it's good for your hair *and* your scalp. This recipe is especially great for fine hair.

2 tablespoons apple cider vinegar
1 egg
½ cup beer! (or an equal amount of aloe juice if you are
    gluten-free)

Combine all ingredients in a small bowl and whisk or stir well. Apply over entire head and either wrap in a towel and leave for up to thirty minutes, or just coat your hair in the shower and then rinse. Don't use very hot water or you will scramble your egg . . . literally. Take the extra beer into your shower with you and drink it. You're welcome. Makes one use.

HAIR PROTEIN TREATMENT

A hair protein treatment is very different from a conditioning treatment. A protein treatment helps build up brittle, damaged hair. It will make your hair thicker and healthier. Sometimes after you use a protein treatment your hair will feel drier, but this is totally normal and will just require some extra conditioning a few days later. Don't use this treatment directly on your scalp unless you have extremely thick, dry hair. Shea butter protects your hair from heat, locks in moisture, and helps with split ends. Greek yogurt has twice the protein of other types of yogurt and will help make your hair shiny and strong. Blackstrap molasses is basically a nutrient-dense sugar. It is incredibly high in antioxidants and will also strengthen your hair.

1 tablespoon shea butter
½ cup full-fat Greek yogurt
1 tablespoon blackstrap molasses

Warm shea butter in a double boiler until melted. Spoon yogurt into a medium bowl and stir in melted shea butter. Add molasses and continue to stir. The mixture will become light brown and will smell delicious. Tie your hair into a high ponytail and apply mixture from your tips to the hair tie. Make sure to soak your hair well, not leaving any strands dry. Leave in for a few minutes or through an episode of *The Good Wife*. Use all within one application. You may need to shampoo two to three times to get it all out, but it'll be worth it. Makes one use for you and one for your husband's hair and his beard (feel free to apply it as a mask to your face, too!). Should not be stored.

DRY SHAMPOO BY SKINNYSKINNY

Clara Williams is the founder of the natural skin-care line skinnyskinny. Clara made natural "cool" way before anyone else was even thinking about it. She happens to sell an amazing dry shampoo that I use and love, and she provided me with a simple version you can quickly make at home! As Clara says, "Most people have cornstarch and baking soda in their cupboard. Cornstarch is great for absorbing excess oils, and baking soda helps keep your hair smelling fresh." Dry shampoo is a great way to hide that you haven't showered because you're diligently following all of my advice, or because you spent the night . . . "camping."

10 to 15 drops essential oil of your choice
1 tablespoon baking soda
4 tablespoons cornstarch
Empty, clean, and dry glass spice jar (with shaker-top cap)

Mix the essential oil into the baking soda with a fork or whisk and get rid of any lumps, then add the cornstarch and mix completely. Pour mixture into spice jar and seal with the cap. To use, just sprinkle a very small amount onto the roots of your hair and comb or tousle through to the ends. Store in a dry place. Mixture will keep indefinitely, and it'll make more uses than you'll ever need, though the scent will fade over time.

HAIR OIL

Hair oil is the opposite of dry shampoo, obviously. It's a great product to throw into wet hair to help you style on the fly. This killer hair oil is light enough that it won't make your hair look greasy, yet it will still nourish your strands. Castor oil strengthens your hair and helps it grow, and macadamia oil is moisturizing and soothing for color-treated hair. It also helps with split ends. It's best to use hair oil on the tips of your hair (not at the roots), so start from the nape of your neck and comb downward with your fingers.

1 tablespoon castor oil
1 tablespoon macadamia oil
5 to 15 drops of favorite essential oil

Mix all ingredients in a bottle or jar, seal, and shake well. Use a tiny bit at a time—start with less than you think you need until you know what works best for your hair. This product will keep for a few months and, if used in small amounts every day, will last you about that long. It can be stored in your bathroom cabinet.

SEA SALT HAIR SPRAY BY HERBIVORE BOTANICALS

Julia Wills started her company, Herbivore Botanicals, in her Seattle kitchen. Now she sells her products nationally through stores like Urban Outfitters and Free People. The products are gorgeous. Here, she shares her amazing recipe for a sea salt hair spray. Sea salt spray is a great way to add volume to your hair and give you a wavy, beachy, summery look. Aloe adds moisture to your hair and acts as a conditioner, keeping your hair strong and silky.

1 cup water
1 tablespoon sea salt of choice
15 to 20 drops of essential oil(s) of choice
¼ cup aloe juice (optional)

Mix all ingredients in a spritzer bottle and shake well. For essential oils I recommend a combination of rose and citrus (blood orange or sweet orange). They are light and floral (a bit of a splurge, but a little rose goes a long way in a spritzer like this). For a more affordable option, try rose geranium with blood orange. The aloe is an optional ingredient but a nice touch, especially since sea salt can make your hair dry over time, and the aloe will prevent that. Sexy!

TA-DA! CONGRATULATIONS. YOU NOW have basically every product you could ever need for a great, natural skin-care regimen. You learned about chemistry, cooking, and beauty all in one place. You're kind of like a chef now. It's exciting, right? I feel the same way! I hope you use these recipes over and over, and continue to experiment with natural, homemade skin care forever.

CHAPTER 8

I STILL HAVE QUESTIONS!

This is where I try to think of every possible question or issue you may have had while reading this book or testing out a new eating or skin-care routine. Since I can't read your mind, I'm including some of the most frequently asked questions I get from clients, friends, and strangers when it comes to how some of the diet and lifestyle changes we've discussed here might impact them—and what more they can do to get ethereal, glowing skin. I've broken this Q&A into three sections to make it easy to scan at a glance: lifestyle, food, and skin care. If you don't see your question here, I hope we get to meet someday so you can ask me in person!

LIFESTYLE

Q: Is getting enough sleep really that important for good skin and good health? How much sleep do I actually need?
A: Sleep advice is like water advice—the answer is you will

almost always benefit from getting more of it. But sleep is a very personal and intuitive medicine. If you're not getting enough water, you might not feel dehydrated. But if you're not getting enough sleep, you're . . . sleepy. Your skin is able to repair damage and regenerate while you sleep. It keeps your entire body energized. Signs that you're not getting enough rest include frequent headaches and migraines, moodiness, and an inability to focus. Your skin may also appear puffy, dull, and saggy.

Q: *What's the absolute bare minimum amount of exercise that I can get away with and stay healthy?*
A: According to the U.S. Department of Health and Human Services, it's two and a half hours of cardio plus two strength-training sessions per week.[26] My personal opinion is that how much exercise you need depends on how active you are. If you walk or ride your bike to work, or you're running around with your kids all day, then thirty minutes three to four times a week is probably great. If you drive a lot and sit at work all day, try to get at least thirty minutes in every day. If you don't love exercising, try adding a mantra that you whisper to yourself to remind you that your skin is getting better every second you're out there moving.

Q: *Since I'm taking control of my health, can I stop going to the doctor?*
A: Of course not. Your doctor(s), and for that matter all other health practitioners, are trained experts with knowledge that you don't have. Don't let the Internet convince you otherwise. At the very least, they are great resources for regular checkups and getting a handle on your

baseline health stats. At best, they can find and prevent illness, help you make better-informed decisions, and possibly save your life. Go to your doctors often, be buddies with them, and ask lots of questions.

Q: What about "alternative" practitioners like acupuncturists, chiropractors, and that massage therapist I met at the park who told me she works out of her house?
A: My clients and I all have had wonderful results with alternative medicine, and many treatments can be great for your skin. I generally recommend doing some research before going to an alternative practitioner—a referral from a friend is a great place to start, but do a little research as well: go online and find out more about his or her background. And remember that, like with a doctor, just because you don't love the practitioner doesn't mean you don't love the service. Try again with someone else before deciding if a treatment is or isn't right for you.

FOOD

Q: Am I allowed to drink coffee?
A: Coffee is dehydrating, acidic, and contains a stimulant that isn't great for you—but it's also full of antioxidants and is a beloved ritual for many people. If you like a cup o' joe once in a while because you think it's delicious or because it gives you a boost, go for it. Just be sure you drink a lot of water to combat its dehydrating effects.

A lot of my clients use it as an energy crutch because their lives are too busy, their diets aren't wholesome enough to provide energy, or they're not getting enough sleep. If this is the case for you and you're relying on coffee just to get through the day, please try to cut back. Exercise more, sleep more, and eat more nutritious foods. Swap in different types of tea when you can, which also offer a variety of antioxidants.

Q: I know you said alcohol is not great, but come on. What about red wine? Isn't it supposed to be good for you?
A: The buzz-worthy nutrient that prompted all of that good press around red wine a few years ago is called resveratrol, which is found in the skin and seeds of grapes. Are you going to rush to the store tonight to buy grapes? I didn't think so. Resveratrol can also be bought in supplement form, if you are interested in the health benefits alone. But that's not why you're pouring yourself a glass of Bordeaux at the end of a long day. Ice cream contains calcium. You're probably not eating it because you want strong bones.

As I've said, you are an adult, and you get to decide how much alcohol you drink—but from a health and skin perspective, less is more. Yes, some health benefits have been linked to drinking different types of alcohol, including wine. Sadly, this doesn't justify opening a new bottle every night.

Q: Will digestive enzymes give me diarrhea?
A: No. They are not laxatives. They will help make you more regular, but in a natural, gentle way—not in a stimulant-laxative type of way. If you do get diarrhea, it is the result of something you ate and should not be eating.

Q: Why is home-cooked food so much better for me than restaurant food? Aren't they just cooking the same basic recipes I am . . . but better?
A: Restaurant food is indeed delicious, and it's partially because restaurants use a lot of ingredients and preparation methods that make food taste delicious: sugar, salt, oils, deep frying, etc. Not to mention the gargantuan portion sizes you get at most places. A restaurant meal typically has significantly more calories and ingredients than what you cook at home. So cook when you can, and when you do go out, look for places that advertise the quality of their ingredients—organic veggies, grass-fed meat, wild-caught fish, and so on. Any good chef will let high-quality ingredients be the star of the plate.

Q: What's the difference between sodium and salt, and do I really need to use sea salt? What about iodine—isn't that something I need that I get from table salt?
A: Table salt and sea salt both contain sodium, though sea salt contains slightly less sodium than table salt, and I think it tastes better. Table salt is generally more processed, and it does contain more iodine (added in chemically) than sea salt—it could be a good choice if you are iodine deficient or have thyroid issues. If you are buying sea salt, make sure to do a little research and find a good one (we love Maine Sea Salt and use it in our S.W. Basics Exfoliant!).

Q: How come you didn't talk much about grains in your food section?
A: Grains are so controversial, and everyone is looking for the perfect yes-or-no answer—but I don't feel that strongly

about them. Whole grains like brown rice, wild rice, quinoa (technically a seed), whole wheat, etc., are, in my opinion, all really good for you. They are full of nutrients and fiber. Processed grains are not. If you like grains, I say eat them. If you don't like them or you've discovered while you were food journaling that your body doesn't like them, don't eat them.

SKIN CARE

Q: Are you absolutely, completely, totally positive that putting oil on my face will not clog my pores? Would you bet your life on it?
A: I am absolutely, completely, totally positive. The anti-oil craze comes from confusion. Back in the day, when people's skin began reacting to all the nasty petroleum oil (also known as "mineral oil") in commercial products, companies began to market their products as "oil-free" rather than "gasoline-free," as they should have. The result is your fear of oil. In fact, many companies are now using synthetic oils in oil-free products, and even mineral oil still runs rampant (like in your Vaseline). Natural oils do not clog pores, they feed them.

Q: Talk to me about the term non-comedogenic. Should I avoid products that don't have this word on the label?
A: No, because it is a made-up marketing term whose use is unregulated, which therefore renders it meaningless. Some ingredients, often synthetic, clog almost everyone's pores. Some ingredients clog only some people's pores. Identify the ingredients causing you problems and stop using them. That's all there is to it.

Q: I'm wearing SPF 100 inside my house at night right now. That's what I should be doing, right?
A: No, but I understand why you're scared. Skin cancer is terrifying. If you are more comfortable wearing sunscreen every day, that's totally fine. Just get your vitamin D levels checked regularly, and choose your sunscreen carefully. That means looking for a product with no nanoparticles (these penetrate your skin and are highly toxic) or oxybenzone. Do some research online, especially on ewg.org/skindeep, and choose sunscreens with a safe rating (this is especially important for sunscreen you use on your children!).

Q: I have body acne. Is it caused by the same things as my face breakouts, and should I be treating it differently?
A: Body acne is indeed caused by the same things as facial acne. And if you break out on your face, you are also more likely to break out on your body. In other words, usually they happen together. What a bummer, right? Treat it the same as you would a breakout on your face—use a high-quality cleanser or soap, try a dash of sea salt or baking soda, and don't forget to moisturize.

Q: How do I know the difference between a detox skin symptom and a bad reaction?
A: This one is a little bit tricky because it's very personal. I will say that a bad reaction is usually much worse and lasts much longer than a detox symptom. So exfoliating may make you break out for a few days or even a week, but it will not make you break out forever. A bad ingredient that you continue to use will. A negative reaction will occur everywhere that a product or ingredient has touched your

skin. If you are unsure, err on the side of bad reaction and stop using whatever you're using.

Q: One time I used olive oil and broke out and got bright red and stayed that way for three days. I'm terrified of natural ingredients now. How do I get over that?
A: By not grouping "natural" ingredients in one big category. Would you stop using mascara because one didn't work for you? Or lipstick? Or toothpaste? No, you would stop using that brand and try a different one. Don't let that olive oil experience ruin it for all the others.

Q: I have a hard time digesting gluten. Is there anything I should do differently when I'm making my DIY products?
A: There's very little gluten in the recipes, but when a recipe calls for anything that worries you, swap in your favorite gluten-free versions (I love Bob's Red Mill).

Q: I have terrible skin and feel like I've tried everything in this book but nothing helps. What now?
A: The next step is to have a one-on-one with a professional. Visit your doctor or dermatologist, see a naturopath, schedule a consultation with a nutritionist, hire a holistic health coach. You may need the perspectives of a few different health practitioners to solve the problem, but don't worry, if you keep looking for the answer, you will find it! I promise.

CONCLUSION:
YOU DID IT!

I n my dream world, a healthy lifestyle is just that: *one* healthy lifestyle. One among billions. If you're like me, you can't help but read celebrity gossip magazines that promise that you'll look exactly like some gorgeous movie star if you just follow her diet, her exercise plan, and her skin-care routine. You try to follow it perfectly, and what happens? That's right, you stay looking exactly like yourself. Well, of course you do! Following someone else's routine isn't going to work the same for you as it does for them, and it's most definitely not going to turn you into them.

It's important that we all learn not to box ourselves into other people's definitions of healthy living. We have categories like "vegetarian," "Paleo," "raw," and "gluten-free," but these neat categories often distract us from finding what's best for us. Terms like these are actually identities masquerading as diets. They're tools people tend to use to fit into a specific social group, and they distract us from the fact that we all have completely unique bodies with completely unique needs.

The only way to create your own individualized picture of wellness is to commit to finding the ideal version of your personal everyday health. That requires being really in tune with your body's (sometimes subtle) symptoms, being honest with yourself about your behaviors, and being aware of the correlations between the two. We must come to see our health as *our* responsibility—not the responsibility of our doctors or our government or the chefs at our favorite restaurants.

The same is true for skin care. I'll be the first to argue that the FDA and the industry's major players have let the average customer down in a huge way. But it's still *my* responsibility to take care of myself while I force big corporate dinosaurs to change with the ways I choose to spend (or not spend) my dollars.

My client Laura offers a great example of what I think it looks like to take charge of your personal wellness. She was a huge skeptic when I first met with her, but once she became more informed about her health and how her habits impacted her skin, she experienced dramatic results. I'll let her tell you the story in her own words . . .

When I came to Adina, I thought of myself as being really healthy and really informed. Big lightbulbs went off when I started keeping a food and product journal: I didn't really realize I was having three cups of coffee *every day*. Or eating so much soy.

Then I wrote down all the products I was using, and when I looked at the list, I was a little shocked. It added up to a lot of products that I kept mixing up. When one miracle face wash didn't do the trick, I'd switch to the next, but kind of keep everything else in rotation.

Now I still wash my face every day, but I'm using mânuka honey, jojoba oil, and a little castile soap if I've been wearing a lot of makeup or sweating. I'm also into cleansing with a mix of castor oil and thyme essential oil, and I love coconut oil for body lotion. Using these products has made a huge difference. I no longer have oily skin. I am maybe still a product junkie, but these days I'm mixing up concoctions myself.

I've settled into a happy eating routine, too. Dairy and wheat seem to trigger breakouts for me (baked goods especially!). It took me a while to stop missing dairy, but I'm finally there, because I've found enough alternatives I like. It feels too hard to never eat wheat or white flour, so I just pay attention to how much I'm eating. I also notice that I have great skin when I'm cooking more.

Other people put on weight as soon as they eat a muffin. For me, bad eating would always trigger a breakout. I used to ask "Why me?" but I have come to be grateful for my skin, because I really feel that I am altogether healthier now and more in tune with my body because of the distress signals it was sending me.

MOST OF US FIND health and skin care stressful and confusing because we're always trying to fit what *our* body does into someone else's system. But once you become attuned to your individual body and your individual skin, no matter what your personal routine looks like, there's no reason for it to be stressful or confusing. That's why I wrote this book, because I want you to use all of this information to get to know yourself really well, and then I want you to stop stressing about it once and for all.

My last and final plea to you is this: please remember how empowering it is to take care of yourself. Remember that when you feel good, your whole life gets better. Remember that when you make choices that are good for you, they are also good for everyone around you and for the planet. Remember that your features make you *you*, and remember that you are awesome.

ACKNOWLEDGMENTS

This book was possible because of every person who has supported me from the second I decided I loved attention. Thank you to all of you, and especially to:

Adam Poor, who deserves a writer credit for this book and really for my whole life. Thanks for helping to shape me into a functional, happy human being.

Anca Grigore, for teaching me an HSP can still be HBIC. Kayla Simpson, for being the third puzzle piece to our crazy little universe.

Elana Bowsher, truly an angel sent from a magical place to save us. Dalton Abbott, for being the most genuinely supportive and kind human to ever exist.

Jessica Assaf, for causing good things to happen from the moment we met, and for believing in me more than I have ever deserved. MacKenzie Smith, for helping make us cool and for being so sweet while you did it. Jess Blackman, for being more worth stalking than I could have ever imagined. Sona Banker, Julia Sweeney, and Leslie Hollingsworth, for joining me right as things got really crazy.

Libby Vanderploeg, for being a genius and a peach. I love your work and what you did for this book. So lucky to have found you right in my backyard!

Lindsay Edgecombe, this book would not exist without you. Thank you for being a true friend. You helped me believe I could actually do this, a million different times.

Julie Will, for making me sound like a real writer, and for putting up with all of my annoying shenanigans. Sydney Pierce, for calming me down over and over. Leigh Raynor and Christine Choe, for loving on this project and helping me find my readers!

Katie Klencheski and the team at SMAKK Studios, for creating a brand that makes people swoon.

Megan Shockney, for making us famous. Eden Grimaldi, Brittany Rupp, and the team at MediaCraft, for helping us grow up.

Mona Salib, for standing by me throughout the years, and for being a guiding light and an inspiration. Samer Altaher, for making us feel legit and loved from day one.

Andy Secunda, the greatest friend and mentor anyone could ever ask for. Kate Hess, for cheering me on (and commiserating) while we tan.

Rachel Siegel, for literally showing me my future and making me pursue it, and then showing up without being asked every time I needed help. Brad Jenson, for getting really into skin care for us.

David Borman and Saskia Hildebrandt, for being my life role models.

Ryan Nagel, for sending love from afar, always in the perfect moments. Jodi Nagel, for being our number one Florida booster.

Heather and Michael Terry, for your support, guidance, and patience. Lots and lots of patience.

Zak Normandin, for teaching me how to keep my cool under massive amounts of pressure. Even though you look better doing it.

Larry Betz, Jesse Gonzalez, Ashley Koff, Megan Mc-Grane, Andy Bellatti, Laurie Brodsky, Jennifer Mielke, Frank Lipman, Sarma Melngailis, Jordan Pacitti, Rachel Winard, Clara Williams, Julia Wills, the Environmental Working Group, and Dr. Carlos Charles, for help with research and quotes, often under a tight deadline.

Maddie Gubernick, Liza Henowitz, and Val Volkov, for help with recipes and research.

Sarma Melngailis, Katie Quilligan, Amelia Stocker, Tiffani Barton, Karen McDermott, Brittany Travis, Neal Harden, Anita Shepherd, Shaun Boyte, Elizabeth Sorrell, Dan Berger, Katherine Jaeger-Thomas, Jacob Thomas, David and Saskia, Rachel and Brad, Lucas O'Neill, Arianne Keegan, Ali Accarino, Ilana Diamond, Jen Koehl Uphues and Chris Uphues, Melissa Goldstein, Josephine Cameron, David Goldberg, and many more, for being wonderful humans who have supported S.W. throughout the years without anything to gain.

Pamela and Michael Poor, for making me feel like family, and for treating our wild ride like the coolest thing ever. Daniel Poor, for being a part of the ride with us.

And last but definitely first in many ways, Mom, for encouraging me to embrace who I am from day one, and for making me feel like it's the best way to be.

NOTES

1. "Acne: Diagnosis, Treatment, and Outcome." American Academy of Dermatology. Accessed August 17, 2014, http://www.aad .org/dermatology-a-to-z/diseases-and-treatments/a---d/acne /diagnosis-treatment.
2. "Psoriasis: Who Gets and Causes." American Academy of Dermatology. Accessed August 17, 2014, http://www.aad.org /dermatology-a-to-z/diseases-and-treatments/m---p/psoriasis /who-gets-causes.
3. "What Is Eczema?" American Academy of Dermatology. Accessed August 17, 2014, http://www.aad.org/dermatology-a -to-z/for-kids/about-skin/eczema-itchy-skin/what-is-eczema.
4. Wilhelm Stahl et al. "Carotenoids and Carotenoids Plus Vitamin E Protect Against Ultraviolet Light–Induced Erythema in Humans." *The American Journal of Clinical Nutrition* 71 no. 3 (2000): 795–98.
5. Rob Dunn. "Human Ancestors Were Nearly All Vegetarians." *Scientific American.* July 23, 2012. Accessed September 24, 2014, http://blogs.scientificamerican.com/guest-blog/2012/07/23 /human-ancestors-were-nearly-all-vegetarians/.
6. Amy Paturel. "Does Your Diet Fit Your Genes?" IDEA Health and Fitness Association. Accessed August 17, 2014, http://www .ideafit.com/fitness-library/does-your-diet-fit-your-genes-0.

7. "Don't Count Dad Out," University of Utah Health Sciences. Accessed August 17, 2014, http://learn.genetics.utah.edu/content /epigenetics/nutrition/.

8. Amit Mohan et al. "Effect Of Meditation On Stress-Induced Changes In Cognitive Functions." *The Journal of Alternative and Complementary Medicine* 17 no. 3 (2011). Accessed September 20, 2014, http://online.liebertpub.com/doi/abs/10.1089/acm.2010.0142.

9. Abiola Keller et al. "Does the Perception That Stress Affects Health Matter? The Association with Health and Mortality." *Health Psychology* 31 no. 5 (2012): 677–84.

10. Bas Verplanken and Suzanne Faes. "Good Intentions, Bad Habits, and Effects of Forming Implementation Intentions on Healthy Eating." *European Journal of Social Psychology*. Accessed September 20, 2014, http://onlinelibrary.wiley.com/doi/10.1002/(SICI)1099 -0992(199908/09)29:5/6%3C591::AID-EJSP948%3E3.0.CO;2-H /abstract.

11. See Tiny Habits Web site: http://tinyhabits.com/.

12. Gretchen Reynolds. "Younger Skin Through Exercise." *The New York Times*. April 16, 2014, http://well.blogs.nytimes .com/2014/04/16/younger-skin-through-exercise/.

13. "Exercise and Depression." Harvard Health Publications. Accessed August 17, 2014, http://www.health.harvard.edu /newsweek/Exercise-and-Depression-report-excerpt.htm.

14. See United States Department of Agriculture Web site: http://ndb .nal.usda.gov/ndb/foods.

15. S. Sinatra et al. "The Saturated Fat, Cholesterol, and Statin Controversy: A Commentary." *The Journal of the American College of Nutrition* 33 no. 1 (2014): 79–88.

16. Graham A. Rook. "Regulation of the Immune System by Biodiversity from the Natural Environment: An Ecosystem Service Essential to Health." *Proceedings of the National Academy of Sciences of the United States of America* 110 no. 46 (2013): 18360.

17. "FDA Authority Over Cosmetics." U.S. Food and Drug Administration. Accessed August 19, 2014, http://www.fda.gov /Cosmetics/GuidanceRegulation/LawsRegulations/ucm074162.htm.

18. "About the Personal Care Products Council." Personal Care Products Council. Accessed August 19, 2014, http://www. personalcarecouncil.org/about-us/about-personal-care -products-council.

19. "Letter to the Personal Care Products Council and Independent Cosmetics Manufacturers and Distributors Concerning the Proposed Draft Legislation." U.S. Food and Drug Administration. Accessed August 19, 2014, http://www.fda.gov /aboutfda/centersoffices/officeoffoods/cfsan /cfsanfoiaelectronicreadingroom/ucm388296.htm.

20. "Hypoallergenic Cosmetics." U.S. Food and Drug Administration. Accessed August 19, 2014, http://www.fda.gov /cosmetics/labeling/claims/ucm2005203.htm.

21. "Talc." U.S. Food and Drug Administration. Accessed August 19, 2014, http://www.fda.gov/Cosmetics/ProductsIngredients /Ingredients/ucm293184.htm.

22. "Hope and Hype in a Bottle." Green Products Alliance. Accessed August 19, 2014, http://www.greenproductsalliance.com /pressroom.html.

23. "Hope and Hype in a Bottle." Green Products Alliance. Accessed August 19, 2014, http://www.greenproductsalliance.com /pressroom.html.

24. "Estee Lauder Clinical Trial Finds Link Between Sleep Deprivation and Skin Aging." University Hospitals Case Medical Center. Accessed August 18, 2014, http://www.uhhospitals.org /about/media-news-room/current-news/2013/07/estee-lauder -clinical-trial-finds-link-between-sleep-deprivation-and-skin-aging.

25. Vikas Kapil et al. "Physiological Role for Nitrate-Reducing Oral Bacteria in Blood Pressure Control." *Free Radical Biology and Medicine* 55 (February 2013): 93–100. http://www.sciencedirect .com/science/article/pii/S0891584912018229.

26. U.S. Department of Health and Human Services. 2008 Physical Activity Guidelines for Americans. Accessed August 18, 2014.

INDEX

Note: Italic page numbers refer to charts and illustrations.

olive oil and, 163
sensitivity to, 88
skin cells and, 4
skin type and, 23
sunburn, 7, 11, 23, 26, 47, 83, 139
sunscreen, 1, 138, 213
urban areas and, 26
vitamin D and, 3, 106, 213
sunflower oil, 150
Super-Rich Cream, 180
supplement industry, 38
supplements
  diet and, 38
  good foods list, 103–6
  suggested supplements, 104–6
S.W. Basics, 120, 160, 180, 200, 201
sweat
  change of clothing and, 143
  exfoliants and, 159
  physical activity and, 30, 32
  pores and, 26, 32
symbols, on labels, *131*
symptom-soothing approach, 11

Taylor, Michael, 122
testosterone, 42, 108
third-part manufacturers, 122, 124
Tightening Bloody Mary Toner, 177
tiny habits, 29
toners
  Brightening Astringent, 178
  Clock-Stopping Electrolyte Toner, 176
  Makeup Remover, 178–79
  Tightening Bloody Mary Toner, 177

Toothpaste recipe, 198
topical steroids, 34
trans fats, 90, 111
traveling, 143, 148

unrefined oils, 162
urban areas, 25–26

vitamin D, 3, 105–6, 213
vitamins
  chart of, 72
  fats and, 87–88
  as micronutrients, 70
  sun exposure and, 3, 105–6, 213

water
  alcohol consumption and, 103, 116
  good foods list, 101–3
  health and, 37
  washing face with only water, 155, 157
water-based products, 167
wheat, as overconsumed food, 63
Williams, Clara, 204
Wills, Julia, 206
Winard, Rachel, 195–96
workplace, 27–28
wounds, 168–69

yogurt, 96

ABOUT THE AUTHOR

Adina Grigore is founder and CEO of the all-natural, sustainable skin-care line S.W. Basics. She's worked in the wellness industry since 2007 as a private holistic nutritionist, personal trainer at Equinox fitness, and jill-of-all-trades at the raw-food meccas Pure Food and Wine and One Lucky Duck. She started S.W. Basics to provide products that are gentle for even the most sensitive skin, thanks to their minimalist formulas and whole, high-potency ingredients. It's an approach that has earned Adina and S.W. Basics the praise of celebrities like Gwyneth Paltrow and Hayley Williams of the band Paramore; as well as features in publications such as *Vogue, O Magazine, W, Martha Stewart Living, InStyle, Us Weekly, People StyleWatch, Goop, Daily Candy,* and many more.